"One of Danit's many tal ments. She can spot your physical pain from across a room ánd shift your posture in just the right way to create space throughout the body. *Simply Put* is like these physical adjustments in book form: a clear, thoughtful collection of small lessons and observations, written to be accessible and relevant to all readers, and sure to make big shifts when applied over time. *Simply Put* brims with heart, honesty, compassion, and wisdom."

– Samantha Greene Woodruff, Bestselling Author of *The Lobotomist's Wife* and Certified Yoga Instructor

"For the first time in my life, I laid my eyes on a book that felt like a friend. In a single statement, *Simply Put* is the most penetrating rendition of "Life for Dummies." Every single reminder, sentence, and overview provides tangible mechanisms for life's endless pickles in a way that allows you to feel human during the process. A truly life-changing read."

– Netta De Lagrave-Codina, World Competitive Figure Skater, Coach and Choreographer, Program Coordinator

"*Simply Put* is an invitation to consider our daily experiences differently, take a bird's eye view, remain true to ourselves, and accept the impermanent nature of life. Danit provides the opportunity and permission for us to truly observe our discomfort and vulnerability while making them the stepping stones of learning and strength on our individual paths. Danit's sincere and compassionate writing is as approachable as she is, and *Simply Put* is a gift to all readers."

– Sonya Sanders

"*Simply Put* tops my short stack of essential reads for personal growth and deflecting stress. With concise, insightful acuity, Danit treats us to a wellspring of practical, applicable wisdom. Her precise and intuitive instructional narrative mirrors her gifted teaching methodology. The tenets of her core beliefs, principles, and sequences cultivate a practice of intention, choice, and awareness. Danit's authentic voice resonates with relevancy, inspiring us to explore our authenticity."

– Marie Kimmel, Yoga by Danit Student

"*Simply Put* beautifully bridges the timeless teachings of yoga with a contemporary and pragmatic perspective on life. Rich family narratives, rooted in a tradition of strong and compassionate women, offer fresh insights into daily challenges. *Simply Put* inspires a newfound appreciation for everyday moments and encourages approaching life with curiosity. After reading, I'll never leave a pickle jar half-open and am committed to embracing chores with an open mind."

– Hadas Weisman

"*Simply Put* is a calming resource for managing life's stressors. Danit's wisdom and skill deftly demonstrate how to apply yoga and meditation to approach the world in a therapeutic and meaningful way. It's a primer for life wrapped in a blanket, with a cup of tea, enclosed in a hug."

– Sharon G. Herzog, PsyD, Clinical Psychologist

"I read *Simply Put* in one sitting because I couldn't put it down. I know I'll go back to it over and over for peace, perspective, and life advice. Readers will benefit from Danit's approach to life's ups and downs — building a solid personal foundation that can't be shattered no matter what life throws at us."

– Alexa Fishback, MS, RD

"*Simply Put* stands out as an engaging guide to integrating the profound wisdom of yoga and meditation seamlessly into daily life. Weaving personal reflections with the physical, mental, and spiritual aspects of yoga, Danit invites the reader to undertake their own journey of transformation, self-discovery, and authentic living."

– Dr. Yarden Finder, Psychologist and Mother

SIMPLY PUT

Practical Yoga & Meditation Tools for a Beautiful Life

by Danit Schreiber

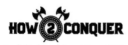

Published by How2Conquer
Atlanta, Georgia
www.how2conquer.com

How2Conquer is an imprint of White Deer Publishing, LLC
www.whitedeerpublishing.net

First edition, November 2023
Ebook edition created 2023
Illustrations and cover design by Telia Garner
Edited by Lauren Kelliher

Library of Congress Cataloging-in-Publication Data is on file at the Library of Congress, Washington, DC.

Print ISBN 978-1-945783-25-8
Ebook ISBN 978-1-945783-31-9

I wish to dedicate this book to my brilliant husband, Jonathan, who put in the hours of support and patience without which this book would not exist.

To my children, Nadav, Netta, and Romi, who are always my inspiration and reason to be a better person and mother.

For my parents, who, even though they are no longer with us, are constantly with me whispering in my ear.

To my students, who have provided much of the inspiration to write this book.

Contents

Contents

Preface

Yoga is the thread that runs through my personal life, from the time I get up in the morning to the time I go to bed at night. Everything I do — cleaning the house, my morning yoga practice, managing conflicts and interpersonal relationships — is based on the concepts and ideas I write about here. This book is a window into my personal practice. It's how I live my own life. This common thread has grown into a pillar that has helped me and my family overcome many of the challenges in our lives. My hope is that by providing this intimate glimpse into my life, I'll offer some inspiration or ideas that'll truly help someone somewhere who is facing their own challenges and travails find their own way to cope and overcome.

Writing this book is a manifestation of daring to be who I am. I've always been loyal to my authentic self, whether or not it was easy or popular, while always respecting others. It's the only option for me. I'm literally physically compelled to be true to myself. There's a price — being myself doesn't always conform to expectations or easily fit into a defined social group. The price, however, is cheap considering the benefit. Being truthful to myself gives me the strength, confidence, and strong foundation needed to cope with the constant curveballs that life seems to fling at us. May *Simply Put* inspire you to dare, dream, and allow yourself to be who you really are with confidence and pride.

INTRODUCTION

As a yoga and meditation teacher, I receive the most joy when I see how people take the tools they learn in the yoga studio into their own hands and make their lives better on their own. The goal has always been to transform spiritual ideas into practical tools that can be implemented effectively in our regular day-to-day existence. I'm blessed to teach a group of students at my studio that has become a strong community. They constantly inspire me with their ability to apply the tools they learn on the mat to their daily lives to overcome whatever challenges come their way.

The tenets of yoga and meditation were created to help people in the here and now. Over time, I've accumulated anecdotes and thoughts that have proved helpful and inspirational to my community. By sharing these stories and ideas with a wider audience, I hope to empower more people to help themselves. If a reader can take one positive idea from this collection that can help them, then it will have been worth all the work.

"I'm Not Flexible"

For many people yoga is quite daunting. Like anything new and unfamiliar, people imagine barriers and obstacles that prevent them from helping themselves.

"I'm not flexible" may be the most common refrain I hear as a yoga instructor. Whether it's a new student or simply somebody who happens to overhear that I teach yoga, people seem to feel compelled to say, "I'm not flexible," or, "I'm horrible at yoga," or, "I can't touch my toes," or, "I'm really stiff. No — really!" or any one of dozens of similar permutations.

My answer is always the same — "So, what?"

Flexibility isn't a prerequisite to practicing yoga, and the ability to touch one's toes doesn't make you a better person.

A student's performance on the yoga mat isn't judged and doesn't receive any points, stars, stickers, or extra credit. Whether or not you can reach the most advanced form of a given pose or the final pose of a sequence does not determine the value of the practice. Yoga's intrinsic value is the process. The ability to reach your toes or not isn't the point at all. I keep reminding my students that they all get 100 percent of the experience and 100 percent of the benefit regardless of how advanced the pose or level of flexibility they reach is. It's about the process.

When you open yourself up to that mindset, you find a wonderful opportunity to learn about the rhythms of your body, your breath, and your mind. With a new awareness, you begin to cultivate new habits and new abilities.

Narrowing yoga to physical limitations such as lack of flexibility does a big injustice to both potential practitioners and the magic called yoga.

The magic of yoga is the positive shift that's happening throughout your daily experience on the mat and especially the shift that occurs over time with consistent practice.

Join Me and Taste a Part of a Yoga Class

Start in a child pose — kneeling, lower your belly between your knees and rest your forehead on the floor. If you feel any discomfort sitting on your feet, you may place a blanket between your seat and your shins. Place another blanket under your feet or knees if you need more support. If the pose causes strain, you can sit in a cross-legged position with or without a prop or any other seated position that will allow your body to relax.

Take a few moments to pause. Give yourself permission to slow down — even for a bit. Notice what you bring today to the yoga mat.

Scan your body, exploring where you feel tension. Don't judge. Don't try to fix anything. Just explore and acknowledge. Take a few breaths.

Notice where you feel the movement of your breath — is it in your ribs, in your diaphragm, in your back, or anywhere else? What movements of breathing do you feel when you inhale? What movements do you feel when you exhale? What's easier for you today, to inhale or exhale? What's usually your pattern of breathing outside the yoga studio in your daily life? Begin to deepen your breathing, inhaling to the bottom of the pelvic floor.

When you exhale, release the breath up and out through the top of the crown of the head. Start to direct your breath gently to all the areas that feel tense or need a little more attention.

Just by focusing your attention on your breathing, you have already slowed down your breath and begun to quiet your mind. There's a calming impact on your muscles and physical body.

Everything is interconnected. When it comes to your physical body, the less you force yourself, the more you'll open up. How do you do it? How do you open up? How can you unlock the knots? Have a gentle, non-aggressive approach; work with your breath, honor your limitations, and be patient. Just breathe. It will come.

RECOMMENDED PRACTICE

FOR A COMPLETE WARM-UP SEQUENCE,
YOU MAY TRY THE "SITTING WARM-UP AND
CENTERING" ON PAGE 179.

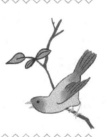

Gentle Reminder

The goal of a yoga practitioner is to get the maximum personal benefit from the practice, not to be the "best," most flexible yogi. In life, as in yoga, it's impossible to be the best or reach the pinnacle of everything we do. We can only focus on doing the best we can for ourselves.

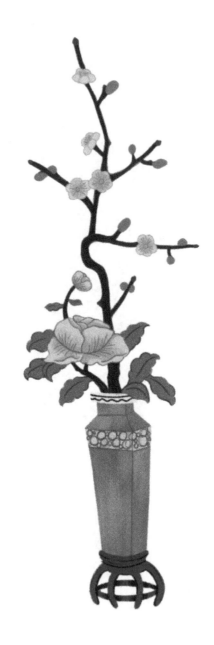

SECTION 1:

CONSISTENCY

Consistency is a commitment to live our lives anchored to a solid foundation. It's a routine, pattern, or simply a steady approach to life that allows us to have a solid, permanent, and unwavering rock to stand upon. Choosing to build a solid life foundation through maintaining constructive, repetitive activities; healthy habits; and a good mindset is rewarding.

No matter how you feel when you wake up in the morning or the surprise upheavals that appear throughout the day, your healthy routine offers a solid, calming place to return to and gives you the solid footing needed to create new opportunities moving forward. Repetition carries weight and creates energy. Like accumulating snow, having a routine builds on itself, creating its own gravity. Over time it builds a steady path that's yours to walk. This consistency spreads to every aspect of your life. In due time, you'll find that you're more effective and efficient in everything you do. Consistency provides you with a framework to build stability in your life.

CHAPTER 1:
When the Earth Crumbles beneath Your Feet

We all, unfortunately, must face great loss and upheaval. How do we acknowledge and grieve our losses while continuing with life and meeting our obligations?

January 2012

I'm jogging on the beach in Herzliya. It's early morning. The day is clear, not hot or cold, with mild temperatures. Great weather to run. My pain and agony are beyond words. I need to keep my regular exercise routine to ensure I keep going without collapsing into thousands of pieces. I know she would do the same. I know she would tell me to do what I'm doing now.

I'm looking at the waves, the same Mediterranean Sea I've known my entire life. The sea seems so strong, so innocent, and free from all pain or attachments . . . just another ordinary Thursday.

A few hours later, I'm standing before my beloved mother's coffin at her funeral. My soulmate, my heart, my inspiration, and my best friend is lying still and can't talk. I can't help but think how much she would have to say now. I saw her several days before — sharp, clear, and totally aware of the situation. She told me that I needed to go back home to my kids.

It had been only a few weeks since she was diagnosed with stage IV lung cancer. Too late for any treatment, it was just a matter of time. It didn't seem possible. We had always said, laughing as we said it, that she would bury us all. Life had a different plan. Back in the US, two days later, I'm already teaching class again. Over her grave, I promised her that moving forward I would dedicate every yoga class and the rest of my life to helping people find their comfort and inner joy, if only for a moment.

In *The Pocket Pema Chödrön*, well-renowned American-Tibetan Buddhist teacher Pema Chödrön notes that everything that comes together will fall apart, again and again, in a never-ending cycle (Chödrön 2008). In her words,

"The healing comes from letting there be room for all of this to happen: room for grief, for relief, for misery, for joy."

Turning Inward

Imagine you're standing on the edge of a very steep cliff. Take one step forward, and you'll plunge to your doom.

Turning back isn't better, as vicious wild animals have trapped you. You feel absolutely cornered. Close your eyes and take a moment to viscerally experience this scenario.

What did you feel? What impact did you feel on your physical body? What changes did you notice in your breath? How would you describe what you felt in that present, vivid moment? The desire to live, to feel the central essence of existence — how powerful was that feeling?

I find the harsh edges of life are often the most powerful moments in our lives. These are the moments we learn how strong and resilient we can be. These are the moments that clear away the "dust" of judgment, attachment, and desire that robs us of our contentment. We have the strength to find a way to start again . . . from the beginning.

Gentle Reminder

Even as we strive to cope with loss, the world continues around us. Maintaining a healthy routine can serve as a foundation we can build upon and help us recognize our strength and our ability to start again.

CHAPTER 2:
It's All Our Choice

In addition to profound loss, we all face the random bad mood, annoyance, or waking up on the wrong side of the bed that can be as debilitating as a major upheaval or loss.

You wake up one morning. You didn't plan it. You didn't expect it, but you awoke in a nasty mood. You feel inadequate. You feel lonely. You're running negative storylines in your head. Somewhere in your relational mind, you're aware there's nothing to justify this mood. But this mood feels like goo stuck to your body — it just won't loosen its grip. You feel as if your body is broken into thousands of small pieces.

The house is quiet; everyone else is still sleeping. You allow yourself to go to your yoga mat. Lying down in savasana, you feel as if you sank to the bottom of the ocean. You imagine the sandy bottom. You give in to the feelings. You surrender. You ask for help. The armor, the effort to hold it together all the time, the obligation to be cheerful and positive, has cracked and melted away. You lie there raw and exposed.

You pause. You know that harsh emotions are a part of the whole, part of life. Resisting them, denying them is an act of aggression toward yourself. These are moments of self-teaching. With all the pain, there's also tenderness.

You know that suffering is an inevitable condition for all human beings, so say the Buddhist teachings. Everyone suffers, no matter their specific situation. You must appreciate how lucky you are to be aware, to be able to pause and notice what's happening. You can find the courage to meet things as they are.

Or, you can be trapped, finding ways to deny and distract from the harsh sensations that come up. They could take the form of loneliness, anger, anxiety, sadness, jealousy, boredom. The list is long. Right away, you look to solve or fix the sensations and find comfort again by giving in to habitual patterns of reacting, falling back into well-worn, preordained lines of thinking and doing.

It's early, and you're on the yoga mat. This time, you allow yourself to be with the harsh sensations. You become a bit more familiar with them. You get a bit closer to the sensations and observe them. You close your eyes. I ask you to feel the sensations in the body.

Where are they located? What shape do they form? What color? You stay with the sensations for a few moments, awake and aware, coming back to your involuntary breath. It burns you, you feel the pain, and it becomes a tangible object.

Now imagine that the tangible form of your pain leaves your physical body. You still hold the pain, grabbing the leash tied to it. The pain is there, but out of your body. You've separated from it.

What impact does removing the pain have on your breathing? Do you feel the tension in your body lessen? What of your mind? Do you feel a difference?

Take a few moments to relax with the new refreshing feeling. Cultivate it. There's no need to take back the pain. It's out, therefore it can't haunt you or rule you. Hug your knees toward your chest. When you're ready, roll onto your body's right side, moving into fetal position. Press your hands against the ground to sit upright. Take a deep breath into your heart. Exhale.

Start your day anew.

Gentle Reminder

Having a routine which we consistently adhere to can help us manage our moods and prevent them from controlling us or becoming debilitating. Possessing the discipline to stick to our healthy routines gives us the ability to detach from our negative emotions, so they don't prevent us from functioning.

CHAPTER 3:
Giving, Contentment, and Hoppla Hopp

We're often asked to cope with huge, unexpected change and loss, but how we react to them is up to us.

The 1930s, Center of What is to Become Israel

It's a very hot midsummer day, probably above ninety degrees Fahrenheit with choking humidity. The breeze from the Mediterranean doesn't help much. She's filling mattresses with hay, one after the other. Tedious work. Sweat is pouring from her armpits. She's not complaining; she's right there in the element of doing — present.

My grandmother, Pesia, and her husband emigrated from Riga, Latvia, to help found Kibbutz Shefayim. A city girl and medical student from Riga had to transform herself into a farmer living in the most basic conditions. She taught herself how to like tomatoes. She used to hate them — couldn't stand the taste. Now she eats them gladly.

It was the acceptance of her new reality without resentment. Hunger certainly helped, but she had the gift of presence no matter the circumstance. As a young girl, she used to walk on icy roads to get to school. She was studying at medical school in Latvia before she left everything behind and made Aliyah, the immigration to Israel, to establish the kibbutz. They started from scratch and made something out of nothing.

Looking back, there was a clear pattern. In these early days, she healed a sickly girl named Sarah. Her albinism ill-suited for the harsh sun of Israel, everyone called her "White Sarah." Pesia fed the near-death girl gently with tender hands and patience — a spoonful of food and then another. Sarah survived.

In Pesia's later years, from her early seventies until her mid-eighties, even after losing her husband, she always found herself caring for a friend her own age. There was a never-ending series of peers to look after. When one would pass, she would find herself caring for a new one. She outlived them all.

A few weeks before she died, she still walked with me, bringing a basket of plums to make sure we had food. She was one of my best friends.

My other grandma, a gorgeous beauty who didn't share the same approach to life, used to always say, "Hoppla Hopp, chin up, walk one step at a time." "Hoppla Hopp" was her motto. No time for sulking or self-pity, time to face life.

I saw her a few hours after she died. She was beautiful. Her facial wrinkles disappeared. She was at peace and still so present, in death as she was in life.

In *The Places That Scare You: A Guide to Fearlessness in Difficult Times*, Pema Chödrön defines *bodhichitta*, a term that reminds me of my grandma's strength (Chödrön 2001).

> *"Those who train wholeheartedly in awakening unconditional and relative bodhichitta are called bodhisattvas or warriors — not warriors who kill and harm but warriors of nonaggression who hear the cries of the world."*

Bodhichitta is the Sanskrit word for Enlightened Mind or Mind of Enlightenment. It's a person who's motivated by compassion and seeks enlightenment. *Bodhisattva* in the Buddhist tradition is a person pursuing the path toward an enlightened state.

Gentle Reminder

With the right frame of mind, we can choose our attitudes. We aren't solely the victims of circumstance. Our choice of a positive attitude can create a whole new flow of energy and direction.

CHAPTER 4:
Saucha

I once heard the expression, "Torah is not in the heavens," meaning that it's supposed to be a living document for the here and now. The wisdom we can take from Yoga can similarly be applied to help us manage our day-to-day lives.

Saucha is the first element of the *Niyamas*, the personal practices one must observe as described in *The Yoga Sutras of Patanjali.*

The Yoga Sutra is a treatise compiled by the Sage Patanjali. It codified the philosophy of yoga and listed and addressed the first five *Yamas* (social restraints). The five *Yamas* are the basis for the first of the eight limbs of yoga that define how to live a purposeful life.

Saucha is the first of the five *Niyamas*, which are the second of the eight limbs of yoga. *Saucha* means purity, cleanliness — inside and outside.

For more context, see "The Five Yamas" on page 104

Saucha can be applied on the physical plane: perhaps when placing your yoga mat in a straight line in class, keeping a clean work desk, or maintaining personal hygiene. It can be applied to your emotional and spiritual well-being, whereby you unclutter disruptive patterns of thinking that can cause harm to yourself or others.

There's a connection between body and mind, or the physical and spiritual. As they're connected, one affects the other, so both positive and negative energy can flow reciprocally between the two. One mindful effort on one plane, physical or spiritual, can become the tiny pebble you throw in the lake, creating waves that spread throughout the other plane. One positive act can impact your entire being, setting a new dynamic, giving you the appetite to do more. One positive act can shift your entire life.

It's not about chasing perfection and ultimate clean-liness. It's about placing your attention on the task at hand out of respect for yourself and those around you. It leads to inner joy and calmness.

Approach Everything with Saucha

Start with the small, tangible things, and you will find you create more room in your environment and life for bigger things. The effect will radiate to every area of your life, and it will become the way you live — deliberately taking care of things out of responsibility. By implementing *saucha*, you cultivate awareness in every present moment, because every moment matters.

Think about a yoga class. You're on the mat and the teacher asks you to take a yoga block and place it on the mat. You can grab and place the block mindlessly, without any attention. No big deal, it's a harmless action.

You can instead take the other approach. You pay attention to how you hold the block between your hands, where you place it on the mat, with respect. You carry this respect in every moment of your practice. You cultivate a present awareness of your body's sensations, matching your movements with your breath and your internal feeling with the external environment. You respect your fellow practitioners. You respect yourself, knowing your boundaries and how to honor your edge. You stay safe but reach your limits. You reap the maximum benefits from your practice.

Living with Saucha in Your Everyday Life

The question here is not only how you approach things but also how consistent are you in your approach? Are there areas in your life where you are fully aware and responsible for practicing *saucha*? Are there other areas where you lack it?

Pickles Anyone?

Consistency in applying Saucha enables the development of strong, positive, habitual patterns which enable you to create order in your life. I once convinced a close friend of mine that properly sealing the pickle jar in his fridge hermetically every time he ate pickles would improve his ability to close business deals. My friend had a habit of grabbing a pickle and haphazardly replacing the cover. It may sound insane, but it worked. He was more aware of every action and every detail. He became more focused on completing every action to the best of his ability. He learned how to become a "closer." He learned how to direct his energy and mind in the right direction, in all aspects of his life, whether closing pickle jars or business deals.

Gentle Reminder

Habits are a powerful force that can direct our behavior for better or worse. Cultivating good habits, even the most basic ones, can have a broad, powerful effect on our lives. Building a specific habit, such as learning to be detail-oriented, can even affect our careers in a narrower application.

CHAPTER 5:
A Race against Time

In our modern world, we are bombarded by images of the ideal. Companies and people constantly "sell" perfect lives and images, both wittingly and unwittingly. How are we to reconcile this onslaught of impossible standards with our authentic selves?

I recently read an interview with a plastic surgeon. He told the journalist that women were now asking him to make them look like the selfies they post on social media — selfies that were taken from ideal angles to enhance their features, combined with sophisticated filters, and in some cases touched up with Photoshop. The women explained how they can't bear the fact that their appearance in the mirror is so different from the picture they present on the internet. The gap between these heavily edited, non-human images and everyday reality is too challenging to manage crossing. The surgeon noted that this new desire was universal in his practice to patients of all ages. Even young women in their twenties felt the need to impose the fiction presented online on reality. This artificial requirement to present the perfect appearance only grows with age. Women become trapped in a fight against time and reality.

In her book *When Things Fall Apart*, Pema Chödrön addresses impermanence as one of the three truths of our existence. She explains how everything in life and the universe is constantly evolving. Impermanence is a key feature of reality, and we can only be in harmony when we stop struggling against it and accord with reality. Peace, she explains, comes when we can see infinite pairs of opposites as complementary.

To her point, everything that ends is also the beginning of something else. Harmony and peace cannot be achieved by pursuing one goal at the exclusion of another. They're about relating to where we are, as we are. While we can't accomplish everything in life and must prioritize and make some sacrifices, we also must avoid becoming one-dimensional. We can't obsess over one ambition at the expense of everything and everybody else in our lives. For example, our demanding careers may provide our live-lihood for ourselves and our families, but when our career dominates our lives at the expense of everything else, we may sabotage ourselves, our well-being, and the well-being of the people we love. Our wellness cannot coexist with an extreme lack of balance. Our careers, as our youth, are impermanent and fleeting. If we obsess and build our entire personality on a single pillar, we're left with nothing when it inevitably crumbles.

Aging is the manifestation of impermanence. When we remove the societal pressures to appear young, aging is a sacred journey, a key element in the cycle of life. Growing older has built-in beauty, tenderness, joy, sadness, innocence, and wisdom. The question becomes how to best manage the physical changes we encounter as we age.

Fighting a universal phenomenon head-on is setting us up for failure and disappointment. There's nothing wrong with pursuing and maintaining a youthful appearance. There's real value in respecting yourself and working to present the best version of you. The question becomes: how much intervention is right? And what are reasonable expectations for intervention? To clarify, it's a personal preference. There's no absolute right or wrong. The point is to find balance. Excessive external intervention is the equivalent of trying to control the fundamental forces of the universe. It's an attempt to create a small, isolated zone that's frozen in time while stronger forces continue to exert their power all around. Is there harmony in all that? Can something so dissonant with the universe succeed?

Exercise, nutrition, positive thinking, and, yes, some external boosts can help us feel better about ourselves. Trying to be the best version of our authentic selves has value and is in harmony with the forces of the universe.

There is, however, a fundamental dissonance between trying to be the best version of ourselves and trying to become a live version of digitally altered selfies. Staying human and authentic is far more beautiful and appealing than an artificial, wrinkle-free appearance that doesn't exist in our natural world.

Gentle Reminder

We all have the wisdom to differentiate between what's realistic and false promises that are too good to be true. Being able to take a pause and go back to our breath will give us the space to create the conditions we need to objectively evaluate what we are being "sold," whether it is realistic and sustainable, and how to find the right path forward.

CHAPTER 6:
Washing Bottles

At home and at work, we're constantly encountering tough questions and problems that need solving. Paradoxically, we can often find the way forward when we live in the present moment and let go of the pressure to procure answers right away.

Israel, the Late 90s

Our twins are babies, and the work is never-ending. Washing bottles is one of those tasks that constantly has to be done, over and over again. Whether it's the first thing in the morning or the last thing at night, a bottle always seems to need washing. It's constant work. My husband shares that he has his best ideas that lead to breakthroughs at work when he's washing bottles. Engaging in a repetitive activity that has become virtually automatic allows his brain to relax and separate itself from the stress and turmoil of working, studying, and raising children. Freed from strain, he's able to access a bit of inspiration, and brilliant ideas arise.

New York, Summer 2020

The twins are now adults. COVID-19 has been with us for many months and will be with us for many more. We're all caught trying to cope in the midst of a global crisis. The world has changed, and the shift is felt on almost every level.

The depth of the impact is immense and lingering, causing massive collateral damage.

The first few months presented a shocking new reality; everyone struggles to adapt. The current situation is muddled with uncertainty. Some places, industries, and activities are improving, while others are deteriorating. It feels as if there's no end in sight.

How do we find ideas that can help us cope with the difficulties of a seemingly hopeless situation? How can we form the conditions we need to nourish creative and positive thinking?

In this situation, as in many others, science and yoga overlap in providing the answer. Our brains are at their creative best — poised to find inspiration — when we're relaxed, and our minds are at rest. We can't find the eureka moment when we obsess and try to solve a problem by force. The practice of yoga and meditation — learning the discipline to set aside our worries, to be in the moment, to breathe and achieve true relaxation — is what enables our minds to naturally find the answers we seek.

The practice of yoga and meditation can cultivate these abilities the same way that washing bottles helped my husband find his best ideas all those years ago.

Inner Calm

Yin yoga — a practice that targets the joints through holding each pose for an extended period of time (usually three to five minutes) helps achieve this calm state of mind.

> Restorative yoga — a practice that helps soothe the parasympathetic nervous system through poses supported by props where the student exerts no physical effort, can also help create this atmosphere.

In a yin and restorative class, a student expressed her sense of being "totally tuned out" by becoming so engaged with her breath and body sensations that throughout the class, she wasn't "thinking," and she was free from inner turmoil. For her, it was a similar rest to the one that Jonathan had while washing our babies' bottles. When engaged in the immediacy of our experience, we can free ourselves from our racing mind. Resting in a calm space allows us to rejuvenate. That tranquil space, like a magic well, elevates answers and refreshing perceptions on its own.

We all have this ability. We simply need to carve out the time, so we can create the conditions that enable us to access our innate capacity to help ourselves. Consistent practice enables us to develop new positive habits and patterns we can access and return to whenever we need them.

A few minutes of daily meditation, a regular yoga practice, breath exercises (*pranayama*) — these are all tools that can help encourage a positive shift. We enter the door stressed and worried and exit it in a better place. Consistency, however, is a must. The more we practice, the faster we learn how to access that magic well of goodness.

To cope with this crazy world, I encourage everyone to look inside and use the tools you already have to help yourself find the best way forward. We all have the capacity to take a step back, breathe, and reap the rewards of a consistent yoga practice.

Gentle Reminder

We have the ability, intelligence, and foresight to find solutions we need in our lives. We simply need to be in the right frame of mind. We do that when we have the space to create the conditions to do so. Consistent practice during which we teach ourselves to step aside, breathe, and find space is how we can put ourselves in position to experience a eureka moment.

Chapter 7:
Escaping the Twilight Zone

Life includes many seasons of stagnancy and desolation. Reconnecting with a sense of purpose and a willingness to confront challenges can reignite hope.

Mid-February 2021

The ground is covered in deep snow — a white wonderland. The heart aches for sun and warm temperatures. We're about to close on a year of COVID-19, of closures, social distancing, masks, and a lack of human contact. Despite this, there are signs of hope. The vaccine is here, and it works. The holiday surge is beginning to fall away. There's a shift toward healing and recovery. Yet, we're still living under the rules, limitations, and social order imposed by COVID-19. The soul aches to see people and make personal connections that you can't get over a video call. People are at a breaking point. Still the rational mind suggests having patience, staying disciplined, and not making mistakes. Don't slip up with the end in sight.

It all feels blurry — as if we're stuck in the twilight zone.

In a few weeks, spring will be here. The birth of the new year in nature. Beneath the coat of snow covering the ground and trees, buds and seeds are getting ready to bloom.

Under the quiet and heavy layer of snow, preparations are quietly underway for exciting happenings in the weeks to come. Before we know it, crocuses will pop up from under the snow. In the same way, within our emotional limbo we prepare for what will come next.

❊

To navigate these extremely challenging moments, we can take the opportunity to cleanse. We can begin to shed the layers of emotional trauma. We'll dig ourselves out of the piles of stagnant sentiments, revealing the fresh promise of opportunity budding, ready to bloom into beauty.

Cleansing ourselves takes courage. It might be scary because first and foremost we need to allow ourselves to feel. We need to allow the empty space to fill up with all types of feelings, including pain, without panicking. We can use the current circumstances to focus on our internal gaze, shedding the emotions and fears holding us back.

The good news is that facing these difficult emotions gives us a sense of purpose and the sentiment that we're in control of our own destiny.

This sense of purpose can be our roots providing stability and our motivation to endure through turbulent weather. We acknowledge the nature of the world and have the strength and wisdom to work with its power and energy. We're compatible with the energy that envelops us and consistent in our ability to look inward with honesty. It never fails us.

Shedding these layers of tough feelings, we connect more and more to our unconditional selves. We find a place free from external circumstances, a place we define, the eye of the storm whose peaceful energy is unlimited. We feel free, empowered, effective. We find our inner peace and contentment. A spring cleanse — green juice for the soul.

Gentle Reminder

Real confidence and strength can only be developed by facing and overcoming hardships. These low moments are opportunities to turn ourselves around and become stronger and more confident in our ability to cope. Consistent practice and healthy habits are the preparation, the drills, that we can rely on to be able to put down strong roots, even when we're at our lowest, and to come back stronger and wiser than before.

CHAPTER 8:
Vulnerability

As human beings, we can be both physically and emotionally fragile. This fragility may make us feel vulnerable to pain, which can lead to fear and inaction.

There's a lot of beauty in vulnerability. While it's often associated with weakness, it's actually the road to true strength. It's our human tendency to avoid pain that blocks our opportunity to manage that tender, sore spot in a new way. We may ignore it by running away from it every time we feel vulnerable or seeking short-term solace. It doesn't go a long way. As much as we try, vulnerability will eventually hit us on the head.

Pain is there.

Denying the fear we all feel when we're vulnerable is not the road. It's accepting the fear from a point of true power while not allowing the fear to interrupt how we handle it.

Coming with a fresh perception and insight, we can see that vulnerability is a wonderful tool to cultivate compassion, both for ourselves and others. That's extremely empowering for us as a community. By allowing our humanity and "imperfect" selves to come to the surface, we can stop playing the exhausting game of always acting right and looking right. It reminds me of picture-perfect social media posts that are so far from reality. If we only accept our faults, reality is freeing and human. As others are drawn to and comforted by our authentic self-expression, our lives will fill with true connection.

Feeling Vulnerable?

Try the Buddhist *tonglen* meditation. Pema Chödrön teaches us "sending and taking," an ancient Buddhist practice to awaken compassion. With each inhale, we take in others' pain. With each exhale, we send them relief (Chödrön 2023).

"Breathe in for all of us and breathe out for all of us. Use what seems like poison as medicine."

Here, we all share the painful emotion of being vulnerable as everyone else feels it, regardless of their outward displays. Public and private circumstances frequently, conspire to push so many over their edge. In these situations we should use our common travails as golden opportunities to bind our community and find strength and solace in unity.

Gentle Reminder

While we have the tools to cope with many hardships on our own, we can and should seek mutual help and support from others. Fear of vulnerability leads to paralysis. Feeling vulnerable without shame frees us to seek help and overcome.

CHAPTER 9:
Oh No, I Feel Upset

The unknown and the new can lead to confusion and fear, which can then lead to paralysis and inaction.

Imagine you're driving in a strange neighborhood, and you reach a very confusing intersection. Several streets arrive from various strange angles to combine into a mess of a junction. You're confronted by a mass of bewildering, seemingly contradictory signs: one-way street, do not enter, yield, stop, no left turn, and no U-turn. Even Waze can't save you from this mess. You're totally baffled.

Years ago, as a new teenage driver, I arrived at just this type of intersection when taking the road test for my license. I found myself unfortunately driving the wrong way on a one-way street, with the test supervisor riding shotgun. Personally, I attribute it to being a daydreaming teen.

Humans like to know what they're doing and where they're going. It helps us feel in control of our surroundings and protected from traumatizing emotions like fear, anxiety, and anger. The question is, what do you do when suddenly, without warning, you arrive at those unsettling crossroads and are forced to decide your way under totally confounding circumstances?

Find the Right Path Forward

Begin with a pause. Take time and create a buffer between you and your habitual reactions. Instead of a panicked or impulsive reaction, learn how to accept the situation. Accept feeling unhappy, upset, scared, or whatever emotion arises instead of running away from it. Sadly, there's no way to escape the emotions that are welling up inside of you. In the end, they will always return in one form or another. Be gentle toward yourself and give yourself permission not to be the superhero who always manages the perfect response in real time. Allow yourself to feel vulnerable.

That acceptance creates a cushion of relief that serves as the foundation to move forward.

Now you're ready to move into doing, ready to build a new situation. Thoughtful action can be the remedy as it transforms negative energy and enables the creation of a new reality.

Action starts with positive thinking, a belief that you can find a better way forward. Start with the concrete: a few specific, practical, and feasible steps that you can take in the short term, be it within minutes, hours, or days. Take actions you know can make a positive impact and represent a new beginning, no matter how small. Meaningful positive change is usually composed of a series of very tiny episodes. Together, these small actions create a path towards the desired outcome. In Thich Nhat Hanh's *The Art of Living*, he states that we can leverage impermanence to transform a painful situation into a positive result (Thich Nhat Hanh 2017). In his words,

"Thanks to impermanence, anything can change and transform in a more positive direction."

Our actions are the key to using impermanence to our benefit. You'll be surprised at the impact of your actions. A shift happens as a result of the sequence of accepting, facing, doing, and creating.

Just like I did in my second road test, you'll refrain from impulsively driving forward into traffic, take a pause, and find the right path forward.

Simple, though effective.

RECOMMENDED PRACTICE

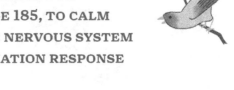

CHOOSE FROM OUR RESOURCE, "SUGGESTED NIGHT SEQUENCE FOR HOME PRACTICE" ON PAGE 185, TO CALM YOUR PARASYMPATHETIC NERVOUS SYSTEM AND ELEVATE THE RELAXATION RESPONSE IN THE BODY.

Gentle Reminder

Denying our emotions doesn't protect or help us. Acknowledging what we truly feel can help us set aside our anxieties and to move forward with a clear mind. Acknowledging truth and reality is a habit that, if practiced consistently, can be a catalyst for finding the best way to move forward when faced with confusion from the new and unknown.

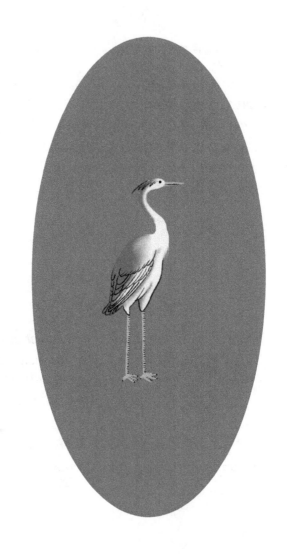

SECTION 1 SIMPLY PUT

1 Create conditions to find inner calm and space with daily routines that direct you to be immersed in the present moment, enabling you to take a pause when you're in crisis, and allowing you to find the calm needed to find a creative solution.

2 A healthy daily routine creates a solid foundation you can return to and use as a starting point to address upsets and crises. Consistency improves your self-discipline and empowers you to be detail-oriented and thorough.

3 Challenging yourself by approaching the edge of your ability is an opportunity to be fully present in the moment. When tested, you must crystallize your efforts and shed all unnecessary thoughts and distractions in order to overcome. Only then can you see the undertakings, start from a point of clarity, and move forward with a fresh, positive initiative.

4 Spreading goodness even a tiny bit goes a long way. Even one positive gesture or kind word can change the dynamic of any situation.

5 Accept that you have fears from a position of strength and confidence. This will empower you to take action and be decisive. It will create a buffer between you and your habitual reactions and prevent thoughtless action in the face of challenges.

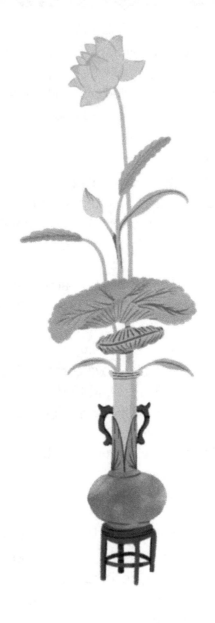

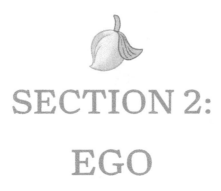

SECTION 2:

EGO

How do we approach the people around us and the circumstances we find ourselves facing? Do we cling to our egos and the stories we tell ourselves when we communicate with people, or do we try to face up to situations we must cope with? Do we see everyone and everything through a filter colored by our own biases? Are we carrying our agenda with us and responding to our own story rather than seeing and addressing reality as it is from a neutral place?

Under all the emotions, insecurities, and agendas that make up our ego, we have an intimate space, free and pure. When we set aside ego and its accompanying baggage, we're unburdened. This unpacking enables us to see the unvarnished truth and conduct any relationship or manage any situation in the most effective manner. Freedom from our own ego goes a long way in improving the results and dynamics of any communication, for all parties involved. Developing the capability to detach yourself from the burden of your own story and rise above old scars gives a fresh new perspective and the space needed to make the best decisions based on an unimpeded view of reality.

CHAPTER 10:
An Unlimited Abundance

How do we measure ourselves and our self-worth? It's easy to fall into the trap of competition and comparison. We then lose ourselves trying to measure up.

We're sitting in the Hayden Planetarium at the American Museum of Natural History in Manhattan, watching a breathtaking space show above our heads: *Dark Universe*.

The show is both breathtaking and disconcerting. It describes the scale of the universe and just how little we know about it. The scale and concept of billions of years and billions of light-years defies comprehension.

Human knowledge can describe less than 5 percent of the matter of the universe. The universe is described as having no center, only an unknown number of interlocking spheres — each representing the observable universe from a given point, each with a diameter of ninety-three billion light-years.

I was caught by that vision. It was the ultimate visual expression of the vastness of cosmic phenomena. It humbles you, being exposed to the vastness and timelessness of the universe. It's beyond the scale of human life — or even the existence of humanity itself.

That said, here on Earth, each individual life can be viewed as its own existence, its own universe — a concept

I find fascinating. The root of the word "yoga" is union, or yoking, from the Sanskrit root *yuj*, to unite.

In the context of yoga philosophy, the union is between the individual soul and the universal soul. There's a simultaneous acknowledgment of these two extremes and how they're connected.

When practicing yoga, I always guide my students to focus their attention on their yoga mats. When a student is distracted, comparing their own body and practice to others' bodies, levels of practice, and abilities, the student loses focus and misses the path that will bring them the greatest benefit. The lesson of focusing on our own practice and what's right for us is a lesson that's as relevant in the outside world as it is in the yoga studio.

Despite the amount of good fortune and comfort, it never ceases to surprise me the lack of satisfaction to be found. Much of this dissatisfaction is the result of comparison. Nothing we have is good enough if someone else has something better. We find ourselves measuring our self-worth solely based on how our "stuff" compares to other people's "stuff." It's as if we're looking at our reflection in a distorted mirror. Our self-worth is dependent on the accomplishments and possessions of others — circumstances we can't control, change, or impact. We bring unnecessary misery onto ourselves, developing feelings of inadequacy simply by having the wrong perspective. There will always be a bigger, better, and cooler house than ours.

Aparigraha, the fifth *Yama* in *The Yoga Sutras of Patanjali*, is about non-possessiveness. In this brilliant traditional text, we're guided to refrain from comparisons that will sabotage our path to happiness and peace within.

The need to compare is a mistake based on a combination of flawed assumptions. The first flawed assumption is that there's a limited abundance we need to compete for in order to find joy. Life isn't a zero-sum game where one person's happiness prevents or limits another's. The second error is the assumption that to be happy we must be at the top of the ladder — that happiness can only be found on the right side of a comparison. The universe is simply too vast for such a narrow view.

The path to inner joy and satisfaction stems from focusing solely on our mats and our lives. By finding satisfaction in doing the best we can regardless of how it compares to others, we remove an obstacle to happiness. Like the vast universe that surrounds us, there's unlimited abundance and endless resources for all our souls.

Gentle Reminder

*We control our sense of self and self-worth.
By focusing on what we have and what's
good in our lives, we can find contentment. If we're
constantly comparing and competing,
we will fall into an unending cycle of
dissatisfaction and unhappiness.*

CHAPTER 11:
A Sense of Belonging

It's a natural human instinct to seek belonging, identity, and community. This yearning can cause us to give up their own identities and selves to belong.

You would be surprised. Whenever I raise the subject of belonging in meditation classes, it always elicits a strong reaction from participants. Throughout the years, no matter the setting or the wide range of people involved, the subject of belonging always touches a nerve as much as it creates common ground. Conversations and class discussions on the topic are always vibrant and lively.

A powerful reaction to the topic is universal regardless of personality type or background. Whether introverts or extroverts — those who are socially engaged or those who are more self-contained — the notion of belonging and all the issues involved consistently draw out strong opinions from all participants. It's always shocking and humbling to see how our assumptions of other people's personal experiences and views are completely different from the personal experiences and views they share with the group. Many successful, capable, popular, and involved people express a strong feeling of isolation, even as they maintain a powerful presence in their community.

The need to feel a sense of belonging is universal. It's instinctual, deep in our psyche. It's the product of our evolution, imprinted in us; it's enabling us to survive, thrive, and build the next generation. Evolution, from our beginning as a species, has required that all humans crave a feeling of belonging to a group to ensure the survival of the species.

Now, hundreds of thousands of years later, we still carry that innate tendency in our modern world, even if the circumstances which necessitated the trait for basic survival may no longer exist. Obviously, we're no longer hunter-gatherers threatened by predators and starvation. We in the US and many other countries are lucky to be part of nations where our survival and rights are protected by law and civilization, yet the visceral need to belong still haunts our day-to-day existence.

To manage this powerful drive to seek belonging and acceptance, we need to understand our personal situation clearly and without bias. This understanding will give us the tools to manage our impulses and the strong emotions those impulses generate, so we can avoid unnecessary pain. Simply knowing that the desire for belonging and a relief from feelings of isolation is universal may bring relief and sense that we're not alone in this struggle. In other words, a sense of belonging.

One of the most effective methods for understanding our personal situation is meditation. Meditation trains us to sit with whatever waves of emotion and impulse wash over us and explore their nature. It provides the space and conditions required to pause and make ourselves aware of truths we never before acknowledged. We learn that a true sense of belonging always begins with ourselves. To extend compassion and love to others, we first need the ability to extend the same to ourselves. The practices of acceptance, non-judgement, nonaggression that help create a sense of community must first be directed inward before we can truly direct them outward.

In her book *Atlas of the Heart: Mapping Meaningful Connection and the Language of Human Experience*, Brené Brown beautifully expresses the idea that we must be able to accept ourselves before we can find acceptance and belonging with others (Brown 2021).

"We have to belong to ourselves as much as we need to belong to others. Any belonging that asks us to betray ourselves is not true belonging . . . Our sense of belonging can never be greater than our level of self-acceptance."

The only way we can feel true belonging to a group, whether at work, at school, or in any social setting, is by being truthful to ourselves. By accepting ourselves, we're able to feel part of the larger group. If we try and adapt to the group simply to gain the acceptance of others without being truthful to ourselves, then we'll never feel an authentic sense of belonging.

The ability to forge real bonds with other people is a powerful tool that makes us all stronger and better able to cope with the challenges we all face every day. Therefore, we must make peace with ourselves. Understand that we already have everything we need to build healthy relationships with others. Once we pass this milestone, we gain the sense of belonging we all crave.

RECOMMENDED PRACTICE

TRY THE "MEDITATION" ON PAGE 188 TO LOOK INWARD AND INCREASE SELF-AWARENESS.

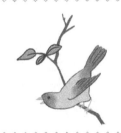

Gentle Reminder

Being true to ourselves is the key to forging powerful and meaningful connections with individuals and the community at large.
The key is to seek belonging without compromising, staying loyal to your true self.

CHAPTER 12:
The Box

We often take what we have in our world for granted, assuming everything will always continue as before. Change, however, is inevitable. The key to coping with change is gathering strength and knowing when to put down our burdens.

Meditation offers an amazing opportunity for learning, exploration, and growth. The practice of meditation can shift our perceptions, impacting our lives in a manner that shifts our reactions, actions, and initiatives. This powerful shift can affect how our surroundings react to us as well. It's a game changer. It reveals our unlimited wealth of wisdom, as if we discovered a secret well of goodness. A space within that can absorb everything, with no bias or judgment, similar to finding a friend who accepts you as you are no matter the situation. Meditation teaches us how to stay still while thoughts and emotions run through our minds. Simultaneously, we absorb the physical sensations ranging from a small itch to achiness. Each time we sit still and meditate for fifteen minutes, we have a different experience. It isn't simple, but the payoff is immense. The practice teaches our body and mind to stay steady — in any condition and through any mood.

To capture the benefits, we need consistent practice. We need to repeat the ritual until it becomes second nature. Once we have built up our practice through repetition and consistency, the whole process feels like returning home. It becomes an anchor that provides stability and safety.

We cultivate new abilities over time in our meditation practice. Meditation is like training in a simulator before flying a jet plane through the turbulent skies of our real-life adventures.

In meditation, many powerful emotions and realizations emerge, and we train ourselves to return to equanimity and clarity of thought by constantly returning to the breath. In meditation we may face a litany of challenges, be it discomfort, pain, anger, or fear — the list is endless. Regardless, we sit acknowledging all thoughts, emotions, and feelings while staying still and returning to the breath.

With time and repetition, we can apply the skills developed in our meditation practice to our lives. We learn to maintain that equanimity in all conditions and situations, seeing the world and people clearly — as they truly are.

Blessed Equanimity

When my mother passed away, my brother collected her personal items and sent them to me in a cardboard box. When I received the box, I was overwhelmed.

I opened the box immediately upon receiving it. Her smell was so prominent, I felt as if I was sitting next to her. I felt buried in her warm arms. I hugged the items and cried, sticking my nose in her coats to try and keep as much of her as I could.

The sensory experience was powerful. I felt the pain of her loss in the strongest, rawest form. I closed the box and hid it in the highest cabinet I could find.

Throughout the years since her passing I opened the box maybe two more times, moments when I felt her loss so acutely that I needed to feel her presence with my senses. Her smell remained for years.

It had been many years since she passed, and for all this time it was hidden in the highest cabinet in the living room. Despite being hidden away, I could feel the box's strong presence, regardless of how much I tried to avoid it. Throughout this time, I set aside the pain and focused on my role as a parent and teacher. I stuck to my routine of not only practicing yoga and meditation, but also learning and deepening my knowledge and understanding.

Suddenly, without warning, I had a gut feeling that it was time to face my pain and release the demon that had clung to me. It was time to move forward. The energy around the box was stagnant, like a raw wound. On a breezy Saturday afternoon, I asked my girls who were at home to join me on the living room carpet. I took the box down and placed it on the carpet in the middle of our circle.

When I opened the box, I waited for the moment when I would collapse, fall apart emotionally, and wail inconsolably. Instead, I was shocked by my reaction.

A river of blessed equanimity flooded through my mind. Opening the box, I took the items out, sharing the stories they carried with my daughters. I saw each item and relived each as they were. I had the courage to look at them, to feel them. My fear no longer paralyzed me.

I had the emotional ability to bequeath the contents of the box to my girls. To enable them to take the past and move forward into their own futures. For the first time I saw my mother's place in the continuation and growth of my family. I moved beyond a feeling of loss that was stuck in space.

As for the box, it's no longer there. After unpacking the box, we placed it in a recycling bin, the cardboard covered with a coating of dust. So much pain contained in a simple cardboard box.

I cleaned the shelf, making room for something new. After years of meditation, I was able to come back to the box better equipped to face the loss it represented. Stagnant energy trapped for years began to flow. The repetition, consistency, and patience cultivated over time helped me face my demons and turn an open wound into a positive legacy I could bestow upon my family.

�֍

Times such as these, when we feel challenged, isolated, overwhelmed, are the moments to find that stable and solid rock inside of us. It's the time to find a sturdy place to stand regardless of the challenges we face, the time to apply all the knowledge we've accumulated from our meditation seat and our yoga practice, the time to put into practice the tools we've developed to manage crises and challenges.

For a moment we may drop into an empty space, a healing space, a space with no physical boundaries, a space where we find our innate wisdom.

Even faced with a terrible reality, we can still be grateful. We can stay open-minded and adjust. We can find the way to be both strong and flexible, just as we are when we practice yoga. We have nothing to lose and no reason to be afraid.

To quote the meditation master and scholar Chögyam Trungpa Rinpoche (Chödrön 2001),

"Hold the sadness and pain of samsara in your heart and at the same time the power and vision of the great eastern sun. Then the warrior can make a proper cup of tea."

> Samsara is the cycle of death and rebirth to
> which life in the material world is bound.

Gratitude for what we have and have had can empower us to manage loss and change. It frees us to be in the present moment and focus on what we need to do now. Gratitude generates positive emotions and a sense of well-being which enable us to function in the most difficult moments.

Gentle Reminder

Consistent practice serves as the foundation that enables us to face challenges. Focusing on the process keeps us from falling victim to our fears and enables us to face our emotional burdens with intelligence and humility.

CHAPTER 13:
The Seer

We frequently carry memories and scars from our past that weigh us down. While they may no longer be relevant to who we are now, it's all too natural to be burdened by them and allow them to hold us back.

Have you ever had the experience of visiting your childhood neighborhood after a long absence? Tons of memories are stored everywhere. Each part of your old neighborhood — a rock, a tree, a park, or even a stretch of sidewalk — contains memories that bubble up as soon as you encounter that piece of your past. Strangely, your memory, what you perceived as a child, doesn't always match what you see in front of you now as an adult. The giant stone wall you remember struggling to climb on as a child barely reaches your waist. In your head and your heart you'll always see it as a huge wall looming overhead. Then you meet it as an adult and are shocked by its relatively tiny size and weak presence.

Browsing through an album, you find an old picture. It's a picture that was never important or central to your memories. You're looking at the people in the photo who were older and more accomplished than you then, but were more than twenty years younger than you are now. Back then, you admired them, but if you met them as you are now, they would have no significance. In the past, living in their shadow caused you so much pain. There were no bad intentions or malice. All of us were simply victims of circumstance. Circumstances generated dynamics that ignited a vicious cycle of negative habitual reactions, which fed a damaging pattern of behavior. Years later, you still bear the emotional scars. These scars are now buried deep, not only in your psyche, but in your physical body. The old scars still elicit a visceral emotional reaction to certain situations, despite the fact your emotional reaction is irrelevant to your current reality. The effects still influence your present-day perception, behavior, and deeds.

Despite how far you've come, these old scars, even now, can rise to the surface and threaten your mental and emotional health.

You mature. You practice self-observation and intro-spection. You learn to separate your thoughts, feeling the gaps between them. You've developed the skill to discern the source of your emotional reactions. You're experiencing the ability to observe yourself as a seer — as a witness free of judgment, prejudice, or bias. You see things clearly, as they are.

Viewing yourself from the side as an objective observer is similar to a *yoga nidra*.

> Yoga nidra is an ancient practice that consists of a guided meditative journey. Practice lying down with the goal of including full-body relaxation and a deep, meditative state of consciousness.

The more you study yourself as an objective observer, the more you shed layers and penetrate the heart of the matter: the unchanging self, the pure witness within.

You can dare ask, is it worth the pain? Is it justified to let old memories and emotional burdens determine how we react, to dictate how we feel? More importantly, does allowing old scars to control us contribute to our happiness and contentment?

It's always a great moment to be able to shed the burden of your buried emotional scars. Become capable of using the wisdom and enlightenment you've developed to help yourself and the people around you. Have a better grip on reality and the ability to cope with whatever we encounter in life. Know we're all swept forward by the river of life into the unknown future, leaving the past behind, but strengthened by the backbone of love and, critically, self-love.

Gentle Reminder

The ability to find space, step aside, and see yourself and your past as if you're an objective third party can help you unburden yourself from the scars of the past and continue as the person you are now creating, a new path forward.

CHAPTER 14:
The Visit

As we return to past places and see people from our past, we not only dredge up difficult memories that can be traumatic, but we return to old habits and behaviors that don't represent who we are now as people, which can lead to regression.

Going back to your roots tests your growth and development as a person in a manner other situations cannot. Familiar people and places dredge up not only old feelings but also old habits and patterns of behavior that are no longer relevant to your life. Returning on a visit without reverting to old patterns is a challenge that can be met successfully using the simplest and most basic of tools — practice.

Consistent training is the key to successful implementation in crunch time. One of the obstacles to consistent training is overcoming frustration. I learned something about this from my daughter's figure skating coaches, who devised a training method to help her foster consistency. They had her track her practice jumps in a notebook. Day by day she had to register how many jumps she attempted, how many rotations she completed, and how many she landed. As a teenager, she wasn't happy about it.

In the end, they were right. Over time, she was able to track her improvement. She had a tool to look beyond the daily grind and see an objective measurement of improvement and productivity. The hard, consistent work at practice gave her the ability to shine in competitions — under pressure, when it mattered.

The principle of consistency holds true for all disciplines. It's very prominent in the military where a rigorous daily training routine is held as the key to success. During my service in the air force, I saw how the repetitive nature of the training coupled with cutting but constructive criticism honed the pilots' skills to the point at which they could complete any mission even when bullets began to fly.

The ability to be flexible and adjust to unexpected, real-life situations depends on developing a solid core of basic skills through solid and repetitive practice.

With consistency, over time we replace old habits with newer and better habits. We develop a new muscle memory. Then, when confronted with difficult and unexpected situations that dredge up old habits, we're able to maintain our equanimity without regressing.

Accepting the New Reality

Years have passed since my last visit to my old neighborhood where I'd grown up. It's been years since I last spent time with my friends and family there. The world I knew has changed. The places and people are familiar but different. They've grown and developed on their own. Generally, there are no bad intentions. There is a gap — two rivers that, over time, have carved two different paths.

Still, it's challenging to return and be confronted with a new reality. In some cases, it was clear that I hadn't returned to a desirable situation. It caused pain. It still does.

Despite the discomfort, I felt I had the tools needed to cope and manage even the most difficult situations. Consistent daily practice of meditation and yoga have instilled the confidence to move forward based on who I am now and not who I was many years ago.

I felt like a disciplined soldier (once again in my life), who's properly trained and drilled to be able to manage any challenging situation. The concepts and abilities developed through meditation became muscle memory. Without thinking, I accessed healthy and constructive reactions in real time, when it mattered.

The first step was acknowledging the new reality. There was no self-deception, no attempt to sugarcoat it. I had to describe the situation as it was in the starkest terms, recognize my lack of control, and accept it.

The second step was the ability to stay with the pain and not run away — avoid impulsive reactions. Emotionally, I felt as if I were holding an intense dragon pose in yin, my heart burning with my hamstrings in an elongated hold. Despite the achiness, I stayed steady and calmed my worst impulses.

Dragon is a yin pose (see "Inner Calm" on page 36 for a refresher about yin yoga). Start from a tabletop position on all fours. Send one foot forward into a lunge. Release your hips toward the front foot. Release your hands or forearms to the floor or an elevated surface such as yoga blocks or a bolster. Hold for three minutes — if you can. Try and stay still while coming back to your breath and body sensations as the anchor that holds you steady. Remember that you might feel discomfort, but avoid pain and exit immediately if you feel something's wrong. Complete the practice on both sides.

The third step was becoming the seer, to have the ability to become a witness, to step outside of my emotions, and to release my attachments and see the past and present clearly.

The ability to detach myself from my own story gave me the perspective and space needed to make the right decisions and find the wisdom to determine the best solution.

RECOMMENDED PRACTICE

TRY THE "MEDITATION" ON PAGE 188 TO CREATE THE SPACE NEEDED FOR SELF-REFLECTION.

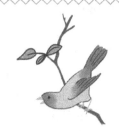

The fourth and final step was having the courage to act based on my new wisdom. Having the ability to see the truth is the foundation, but the value of wisdom is limited if it doesn't lead to action. I had built the courage to free the bird and move on. I could move forward without lashing out, accusing, or causing more pain.

I felt as if I emptied a heavy backpack of worthless and burdensome items. My backpack was now three quarters empty — spacious, light, and containing only essential items. I'm ready to proceed, filling my backpack with wonderful new experiences and feelings.

Gentle Reminder

As we learn to step aside and see ourselves in an objective light, we can also detect whether exposure to places and people will cause us to regress and return to old habits. The present consistency of our practice and our ability to make space enables us to prevent ourselves from backsliding into previous patterns and old habits from the past.

CHAPTER 15:
Pause Please

Disruption in our lives can come from any source. We face challenges in our family, career, and ourselves, but we may also face upheaval and external change completely out of our control.

Spring 2020

It rang like a heavy metal token falling to the bottom of a hole. The weight of it dropped with an ultimate sense of letting go. Watching CNN one evening, the reality hit.

Initially it was something happening far away across the globe, but it arrived, nonetheless. Locally it started small but rapidly escalated, shutting down life as we knew it. What started as a story about a distant land became a once-in-a-hundred-years global pandemic. Its impact will be felt for generations.

COVID-19 is here to stay, for a while. It's not just an episode of discomfort that'll pass within a few weeks. Lots of pain. Lots of sorrow. Lots of unknowns. Fear. Penetrating change. An opportunity to reset, reassess, invent, reinvent. A necessity. It's about survival.

I was raised on my grandparents' and parents' stories: days of immigration, days of poverty, surviving World War II, losing many family members to Hitler. History was told in person, from personal experience. The new life as opposed to the old life. When things fell apart — and they did fall apart for them — they rebuilt their lives from scratch, all over again.

I admired it and felt the lagging effects of their history and their generation while growing up. However, it was someone else's story.

And here we are, having encountered the pandemic, with a massive impact on each one of us. It isn't only about what's currently happening. It's the fact that things will change for good on many levels. The ground is turning upside down. A real vacuum has been created, a tremendous opportunity for exploring new ways and methods of survival. New priorities have emerged for us humans that have basically stayed the same for thousands of years.

The Yoga Sutras of Patanjali describes a practice called *Ishvara Pranidhana*. *Ishvara* is a Sanskrit word that can be translated to mean supreme or God. *Pranidhana* means to dedicate, devote, or surrender (Satchidananda 1990).

"Ishvara Pranidhana involves surrendering oneself to God, in order to reveal the soul. It leads to inner peace, answering the deepest need of mankind, and brings fulfillment of the soul. Inner peace is the absence of internal and external conflict . . . the mind is undisturbed by mundane desires; neither is it and is not shaken by circumstances. There is harmony in the soul as it rests in the Divine."

In *Light on Yoga*, B.K.S. Iyengar explains, Ishvara Pranidhana is an act of devotion (Iyengar 1979).

"It involves humility and love. Surrender of the self means giving up egotism, the sense of the "I" — the smaller or selfish self. The subjective involve-

ment in "I see," "I want," "I do," must be shed so that actions do not disturb the inner being . . . the practice of yoga becomes more important than the person performing it. So that the ego is subdued . . . the practice of yoga becomes an act of devotion."

Among the stormy weather, the unpredictable and unexpected circumstances, we have the innate ability to find the peace. By accepting our humanity, our vulnerability, and finding our humility, we can surrender. We can accept being a part of something bigger. We can drop our narrow perception and explore something new. After all, we are all sharing the experience.

In letting go we find strength and courage to direct our energy to helping others and spreading love. A part of the whole, we each carry a whole universe of wisdom.

Gentle Reminder

The ability to surrender, to know not to waste our energy trying to fight the wind, to make space and step away from the turmoil and analyze the best way forward despite the latest crisis, are skills to help us to grow in the toughest conditions.

CHAPTER 16:
The Finish Line

It seems that there's always a crisis brewing, undercutting our assumptions and forcing us to reconsider our plans. Whether it's a terrorist attack, a stock market meltdown, a global pandemic, or a war in Europe, something happens that shocks the system and forces us to stop and reconsider how we work, survive, and succeed.

Even in the best of times, managing a family and a small business is a challenge that can wear a person down both mentally and physically. Add the complication of a global pandemic into the mix, and the difficulty rises exponentially. Just surviving day-to-day feels like trying to pass the training regimen of an elite commando unit.

Every day poses a challenge greater than the day before, with no end in sight. The continuous mental and physical strain can break the will of the strongest people. To survive the ordeal, you need to develop the right mental approach.

Adopting a meditative mindset is essential. The ability to set aside the chaos and uncertainty surrounding us and successfully focusing on the specific task at hand means engaging in the present experience and preventing external disturbances from sabotaging our efforts. What are the external disturbances that can prevent us from crossing the finish line? Negative thinking, wasting energy focusing on unnecessary and irrelevant issues, and letting the past and how things used to be all prevent us from starting again with a fresh approach.

Negative thinking is one of the primary methods we use to sabotage ourselves. Feelings of inadequacy and self-doubt are just two of a myriad of negative thoughts that prevent us from meeting our daily obligations. While it's normal for all humans to feel these emotions from time to time, the ability to acknowledge them and set them aside, just as we set aside our thoughts during meditation, is the key to being able to wall them off into a separate entity and prevent them from controlling us and our actions. That ability to acknowledge negative thoughts and then set them aside allows us to function in a clean headspace. Without the burden of negative thoughts, we're able to achieve better results, which leads to a positive feedback loop, boosting our confidence and enabling us to accomplish more.

Energy usage is our choice of how we use the limited time and bandwidth we have. We decide on what, how, and with whom we spend our pool of energy. Making the right decisions on how we spend our energy begins with being aware of and paying attention to how we direct our energy. With our ability to be present, we learn to direct our energy to areas that are truly important, so we can turn our aspirations into reality. Given the limitations of our time and strength, we learn to conserve what we have and spend it wisely, as if we're sailing in a small raft and can only take the most necessary items. Wasting space on a superfluous item might mean we won't be able to complete our journey. We're not robots, and managing our energy is easier said than done, but by simply understanding and acknowledging this concept, we can make better use of our time and accomplish more.

Starting Again

Being (or feeling) unable to start again is a common problem. The first step is always the hardest. As circumstances keep changing around us, we're continually forced to begin again. Holding on to how things used to be prevents us from moving forward and finding creative solutions.

Nothing is fresher than a beginner's mind. Adopting a beginner's mind can enable us to break out of the artificial constraints we have set for ourselves. (See "Chapter 29: A Beginner's Mind" on page 145 to dig deeper into the importance of a beginner's mind.) Past experience is an important teacher but can also limit us to a narrow view of the world and how to act. Awareness is the key here as well. Creating space allow us to discern between important lessons learned from the past and old habits and preconceived notions that blind us to new and better ways of moving forward with our lives.

Amid a crisis, it seems as if there's no light at the end of the tunnel, our "normal" reality has ended, and we must accept that we'll never go back. Despite this heavy feeling, the opposite is true. Life and people are resilient, and history has shown that despite the suffering and heartache, we always come out the other side of a crisis and life resumes. It's crucial to maintain our discipline, set aside negative thoughts, and focus our energy properly. Continue to approach each new challenge with a beginner's mind and don't revert to old ways of thinking. We need to accept, like a soldier in training, that difficulty is a part of our training and part of life. Despite this, we won't break, and we will complete our training and continue on.

Gentle Reminder

The ability to access your beginner's mind enables you to take a fresh new look at a challenge, allowing you to take an innovative approach to an intractable problem.

CHAPTER 17:
Saying No

People often ask favors and make demands without knowing or even considering the effect it can have on us. We feel obligated and even pressured to say yes, even when we know that it simply cannot work.

We often address the subject of setting boundaries in meditation classes. The most common issue is saying no when confronted with a request. Many confess they have a very hard time saying no even when they know that there are clear, pressing, and reasonable reasons to answer with a negative. They'll avoid saying no just to eliminate friction or awkward situations. They'll take on commitments they don't have the bandwidth to tackle or insist on maintaining current ones that are a burden with no benefits. Even as situations and priorities change, people will find themselves a prisoner of old patterns and commitments, all because evolving and moving on involves saying no. The fear of disappointing others or, even worse, facing disapproval prevents many people from making the rational and justified decision to make a change.

This seemingly selfless action of putting others' needs first can have damaging repercussions. Completely sublimating your own personal needs can lead to feelings of helplessness, frustration, and even anger. While being a supportive member of the community is important and has its benefits, you must be honest with yourself regarding what sacrifices you can make to help and when you're putting your own health and happiness at risk.

By applying meditation tools and honesty, we can explore the real reasons we prefer to avoid saying no even when we know it's the proper decision for us. While meditating, we create the space we need to investigate ourselves. We can touch the real reasons behind our actions. While we take on commitments under the banner of selflessness, we may find that our true motivations are in fact self-serving. Our inability to say no may be motivated by a desire to avoid awkwardness or conflict. Our assent is usually a quick fix to save face in the moment, merely delaying the inevitable.

Often we feel flattered by an offer or proposal. The feeling of being needed makes it hard for us to let go. Acquiescing when we shouldn't might give us feelings of importance and self-worth even though we know in the end it doesn't make sense for all parties.

In this case, the decision is driven by ego. Ego is the naughty child that toys with our hearts and minds and can make decisions at the expense of our better judgment. Ego creates a zone where we're defined and driven by the stories we tell ourselves. We create a personal zone where on one hand we feel secure and right, but on the other hand, we're unable to make the right decisions for ourselves.

As we sit in meditation, we're able to cultivate an atmosphere of honesty and clarity where we begin to see the truth behind our decisions. We see subtle shades of gray and not just a stark world of black and white. Suddenly we have doubts about the stories and familiar concepts that we've clung to.

With time and practice our perception shifts, as if we're suddenly upside down in a headstand, and the world seems different. Saying no when it's hard becomes a manifestation of integrity. Saying no allows us to handle the situation from a position of honesty and openness of what we need, of what we want, and of what we're realistically capable of doing.

Saying no when it's uncomfortable is also respectful to others. We say no not to hurt or to deliberately cause harm, but to be honest with people.

We honor people by telling them the truth and not misleading them about what we've committed to doing. We need the discipline and strength to be honest and not succumb to the fear of missing out. We learn in meditation to always start with ourselves. If we can't love ourselves, we cannot genuinely love others. While it may seem selfish, the ability to love and respect yourself gives you the ability to extend genuine compassion and love towards others.

Mantra for Boundaries

I say no because I honor my boundaries. I honor my boundaries because I want to make sure that whoever I touch in this lifetime will receive my whole-hearted attention, my honest assessments, my best intentions, and my best efforts. Honoring my boundaries is my way to honor my part in this world.

Gentle Reminder

Setting boundaries not only protects ourselves but also enhances relationships. We should make space and evaluate whether we can take on an obligation, then deliver the honest verdict knowing that we're doing the right thing for all parties involved.

CHAPTER 18:
An Entrepreneur's Diary

We live in a fluid world where we're constantly battling headwinds and inertia. We need a mindset that enables us to adapt and not be hindered by change.

Imagine a small jet plane. It maneuvers in a three-dimensional space, making 180-degree turns, constantly changing altitude, even executing full 360-degree loops. While the plane turns, climbs, and dives, the atmospheric conditions enveloping the plane constantly change. The air pressure, wind speed, and temperature surrounding the plane change as the plane flies. Just as the plane is dynamic, changing its speed and heading, the external circumstances are dynamic as well. There are no constants, just changing variables.

In meditation, we cultivate the ability to find stillness in the eye of the storm. We learn to relax in the discomfort even as we're thrown out of our comfort zone. We allow harsh emotions and thoughts to come up while we refrain from reacting. We sit with it. It isn't always fun or easy, but still, we sit with it.

We learn resilience and equanimity.

When practicing yoga, we learn to find balance between strength and flexibility. To stand upright in a tree pose, we need to pull the energy inward while extending it outward simultaneously. We engage our core without gripping the mat with our toes. We are encouraged to continue and breathe smoothly while standing on one leg. While keeping our posture relatively still, straight, and even, energy flows through our body and we can sway without falling over. The dynamic situation stays fresh in our minds and bodies.

RECOMMENDED PRACTICE

TRY THE "BALANCING SEQUENCE" ON PAGE 183 TO FIND MENTAL AND PHYSICAL BALANCE.

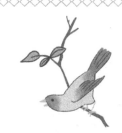

It seems that "calm seas" are fleeting moments of grace that exist between crises. We're constantly faced with disruption and turmoil imposed on us from within in our personal lives and from the world at-large. Whether it's an economic downturn or health scare within the family, the world never seems to give us respite.

In the best of times, running a small business is challenging. The COVID-19 pandemic, however, presented a challenge an order of magnitude larger. Thankfully, some of the limitations of being a small business worked to our advantage. Being nimble, we were able to transform our business almost immediately. We were able to live stream yoga classes within fifteen minutes of a student's request, even before the shutdown was ordered. During the total shutdown, we were able to change platforms and strategies within hours of making the decision. As the date of the phase one reopening approached, we were able to move the studio to a new private outdoor location within days. I was very appreciative of being able to create and be active even during the height of the quarantine.

Being able to create and contribute to other people's well-being in a safe manner helped me keep up my morale and sense of purpose. I considered myself blessed that I had the option of maintaining my business in some form, while others were forced to shut down with no recourse or options.

The extreme situation caused by the pandemic created a unique environment. Entrepreneurs were forced to experiment and innovate to survive. Even as entrepreneurs continue to evolve to meet new challenges, just like our maneuvering airplane, the world continues to change around them creating a never-ending cycle of adaptation.

The changes wrought by the pandemic will be with us for the foreseeable future. As societal norms ebb and flow, businesses will be confronted with a constant barrage of challenges and changes. Now is the time to build a new mindset to effectively pilot your company through ever-changing, turbulent weather. The practice of yoga and meditation enables us to leave our comfort zones, let go of the stories we tell ourselves, and free ourselves to find a new path and reimagine our lives and businesses.

Tips To Consider

* Act fast. Be ahead of the game. Be decisive as if you're a pilot who unexpectedly encounters a mountain crest. There's no choice but to take sharp and immediate evasive action. You flow with the winds around the obstacle and find a new path to travel.

* Focus on continuously honing your competitive edge. Make sure you understand your competitive advantage and put your attention on continuously improving what makes you competitive.

- Think out of the box. Accept the new reality, don't deny it, and accept the fact you have no control over it. Only by accepting the facts as they are, and not pretending they don't exist, can you find a new innovative path.

- Make sure, as much as possible, that you're personally in a good place. If you feel good about yourself and your life, you do your job without distractions from a strong and stable place.

- Be consistent, clear, and authentic. Work from a sincere belief in what you do and knowing why you do it. Know your brand. Work to strengthen it.

- Don't try to please everyone. As reality changes and you're forced to adapt, you can't keep everybody happy. As you evolve you might appeal to different target audiences. Stay focused on your target group. You can't be all things to all people.

- Befriend fear, and don't allow it to take control. Acknowledge that taking risks means you must face fear. Give yourself permission to make mistakes knowing that if you're honest with yourself, you can learn from your actions and use your experience to get where you need to be as a company.

- Stay open minded. Genuinely allow yourself to explore the new situation without preconceived notions. Let go of judgments, stay curious, and learn.

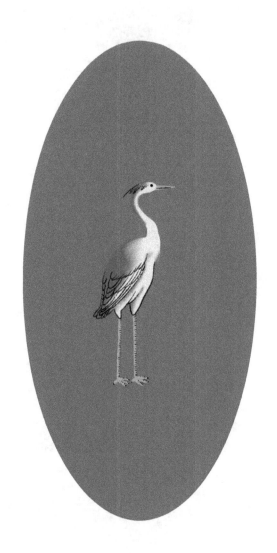

1

The path to inner joy and satisfaction stems from focusing solely on our mats and our lives. By finding satisfaction in doing the best we can regardless of how it compares to others, we remove an obstacle to happiness. Like the vast universe that surrounds us, there's an unlimited abundance.

2

We learn that a true sense of belonging always begins with ourselves. To extend compassion and love to others, we first need to be able to apply these same feelings toward ourselves. Therefore, we must turn inward and make peace. Understand we already have everything we need to build healthy relationships with others.

3

The capability of detaching yourself from your own story and past scars gives the perspective and space needed to make the best decisions based on the present new reality.

4

We decide what, how, and with whom we spend the pool of energy we have. How we direct it will lead to a positive feedback loop, boosting our confidence and enabling us to accomplish more.

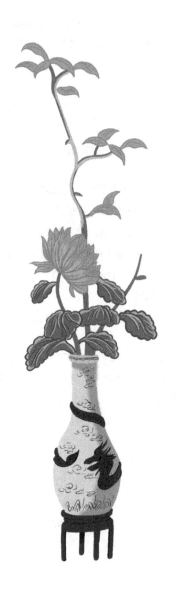

SECTION 3:

IMPERMANENCE

Everything changes from moment to moment. Whether it's a sudden, abrupt change or a gradual, barely perceptible one, life ebbs and flows. For us ordinary people who innately search for the sense of security provided by a comfort zone, it's hard to accept that the comfort zone we're searching for doesn't exist. Resisting the fact that the universe will never let us sit comfortably in a place immune from change is walking a path to certain disappointment. We simply cannot beat nature.

While the external world is in a state of perpetual change, we have a rock of calm and steadiness within ourselves to stand upon. Like the eye of a hurricane, this space is in our core while the world spins around outside. This space isn't a comfort zone where we can retreat. Instead, it's a tranquil place we can use to take a pause, take a breath, and see the world change around us. It's a place where we can make wise decisions on how best to cope with new challenges and changes that are constantly appearing and evolving. When managing the stormy waves of life, we can cultivate a strong core that allows us to ride with the waves and navigate intelligently rather than crash on the rocks and sink. We all have that ability if we choose to access it.

CHAPTER 19:
Puffer Fish

People can often misrepresent themselves and situations in order convey a message or agenda that will serve them. We need to see through other people's motivations to better understand them.

The puffer fish is one of nature's wonders. A puffer fish can change its shape at will. When threatened, it can increase its size by extending its spikes and puffs up by pumping water into its stretchy stomach.

Like the puffer fish, there's a big gap between the perceived display of power and the actual lack of substance behind it. It's fascinating to watch arrogant behavior and wonder what can drive a person to act with self-importance at the expense of everyone else. Those who are blowing smoke create an illusion of strength and size that in no way represents their actual form. A large ego — a cousin of arrogance — is also a distortion of reality. The mind can be an unruly kelp forest where perceptions, ideas, and values are fluid and can grow wildly. It's in this forest that people create their own version of reality. On one side, reality is your past experiences and memories. On the other, reality is your fantasies and worries about a future that hasn't happened yet. We all must contend with the wild thoughts and emotions that grow in our minds. We all face the challenge of perceiving reality as it is despite the stories we tell ourselves. While most of us struggle to quiet our minds, people afflicted by superiority seize their own stories and refuse to let go.

What causes arrogance? It's simply the lack of connection to the present moment. An arrogant person is carrying an agenda wherever they go. That agenda is, "I'm better than you. I deserve success more than you." When a person comes with this agenda, there can be no true communication. There's no ability to be fully present with or aware of other people. That precious seabed of being fully awake, aware, and connected — the ability to be intimate — has been lost.

When encountering arrogance, the best tool is understanding. Being subjected to superior behavior can make us feel inadequate or weak. With understanding however, we realize that, like the enlarged size and the spines of the puffer fish, arrogant behavior is a bluff, a cover for weakness and fear. There's nothing more courageous than being honest with oneself. No self-deception, we meet reality as it is. It takes true confidence to meet and greet whatever comes with an open heart and mind.

It's complicated being forced to manage others' arrogance. In most cases, the carriers are not even aware of the gap between their storyline and objective reality. They constantly withdraw into their story, a comfort zone in which they can deny the existence of any objective fact that disturbs their fantasy. Once we're aware and accept reality, we assess the situation in a new light. We're no longer lulled into the trap. We can elevate above and cope with confidence and a clear mind.

Nichiren Daishonin, a Buddhist priest in thirteenth century Japan, wrote,

"If you seek to become a Buddha, you should lay down the banner of arrogance, cast away the stave

of anger, and devote yourself solely to the one vehicle of the Lotus Sutra. Fame and honor are nothing more than decorations in this life. Arrogance and attachment to biased views are hindrances in attaining Buddhahood in your future existences. You should be ashamed of them. You should fear them."

Swimming in the vast ocean of life, we all have a choice between our own stories or the world as it truly is. To fully engage, we need to drop the attachment to our stories. Only by being fully awake and in the moment can we glimpse the miracle of life itself. It's the beginning of enlightenment.

Gentle Reminder

The ability to take a pause and make space enables us to see through arrogance and defensiveness. It also enables us to keep ourselves from being dragged down into the mud of egoism and to allow us to focus on engaging with life.

CHAPTER 20:
Answering Aggression

We have no control over other people's reactions. We can't always know what's happening behind the scenes. We can't always know what's really occurring in their lives. Many times, a person's reaction may have nothing to do with us.

I was sending out an innocent work-related email with a simple query. The question felt light, harmless, and kind — simply asking for guidelines and clearly respecting the other person's authority as if I were providing a sample piece of fabric to receive an opinion. I didn't expect the type of answer I received. The response was akin to receiving a cease-and-desist letter from an attorney, written in dense, sharply worded paragraphs as if it were a threat to deter an egregious violation of protocol. I felt as if a Rottweiler had been sent to rip my sample fabric into a thousand shreds. I answered with a short "thank you" and an emoji of hands in prayer.

The interesting part was setting aside my own personal feelings and attempting to take an objective view of how I managed the unexpectedly belligerent response. The issue itself wasn't important, so it became a fantastic opportunity to learn about my relationship with aggression. As with any complicated issue, managing aggression, whenever we encounter it, has many facets and angles. This includes managing our own aggression.

Yama

The Yoga Sutra is a treatise compiled by the Sage Patanjali that codified the philosophy of yoga and listed and defined the five *yamas* (social restraints). The five Yamas are the basis for the first of the eight limbs of yoga that define how to live a purposeful life.

The Five Yamas

* *Ahimsa* — Not causing harm
* *Satya* — Truthfulness
* *Asteya* — Non-stealing
* *Brahmacharya* — Fidelity
* *Aparigraha* — Non-possessiveness

The Eight Limbs of Yoga

* *Yama* — Social restraints
* *Niyama* — Observances, rules, and guidelines
* *Asana* — The yoga poses
* *Pranayama* — Breath
* *Pratyahara* — Sensory withdrawal
* *Dharana* — Concentration
* *Dhyana* — Meditation
* *Samadhi* — Bliss or enlightenment

Ahimsa

The yama *ahimsa* addresses aggression. It prohibits any form of what some would translate as violence, defined as harming others or ourselves. This prohibition extends to actions, thoughts, and even intentions. We can learn to apply the concept of ahimsa through our practice of yoga and meditation.

When we practice *asana*, we learn to honor our boundaries to avoid injury. We cultivate the discipline to tune in to our breath and find the appropriate edge for our practice that day. We understand that we can gain the benefit we seek without having to push ourselves beyond the boundary of what's safe.

When we meditate, we learn to let go of our criticism and judgment of ourselves. Sometimes, we sit restlessly for fifteen minutes. Our minds racing, we're unable to place our attention anywhere.

Despite this, we're taught to have a gentle approach, accepting the experience without viewing ourselves in a negative light. We learn to be aware of recurring habits that are harmful to ourselves and potentially others as well.

※

My teenage daughter had a school field trip to an outdoor adventure park. The facility consisted of a series of elevated obstacle and climbing courses, ranging from simple and low to the ground to challenging and frighteningly high in the trees. She was distressed by a group of girls who gathered to laugh at a girl who'd been frightened on one of the easier courses. It was a group of teens that unfortunately found power in putting others down as a way to boost their own poor self-esteem. While distressed, my daughter's ability to take a pause, prevent emotion from overwhelming her, and understand what she was truly seeing helped provide a path for processing the difficult emotions.

When observing the situation from the sidelines, we can clearly see the clique's members focus on finding weaknesses in others as a pure form of aggression. Instead of enjoying their time together at a beautiful and fun destination, finding their edge on the obstacle courses, they waste their time and energy focusing on the weaknesses of other people. Here, and in most cases, aggression is a tool to mask fear and a sense of inadequacy.

In *When Things Fall Apart*, Pema Chödrön poses an essential question (Chödrön 1996).

> *"Every day, at the moment when things get edgy, we can just ask ourselves: am I going to practice peace or am I going to war?"*

The major point is (as always): how we react to aggression is our choice and is under our control. Aggression is everywhere. It shows up in people's expressions, body language, and words. Sometimes it's obvious, and other times it's hidden under all types of camouflage. It's our decision how to react and whether we want to add fuel to the fire or, alternatively, find creative ways to reduce it. Most importantly, we never have to feel trapped or victimized.

We can always find a different route, trusting there are many different paths we can take free of aggression and harm.

Gentle Reminder

By taking space, we can make sure our initial impulses don't dictate our reaction. Instead of focusing on whether we're insulted or offended, we can focus on our purpose and craft our reaction to make sure we achieve our goals.

CHAPTER 21:
Staying Present When It Stings

We're constantly facing unexpected shocks. Life doesn't allow us to stop functioning because of discomfort or hardship. We must be able to continue for ourselves and the people we care about.

We were walking on the beach. It was a beautiful Sunday afternoon, a late wave of summery weather before the temperatures dropped down to freeze us on the East Coast. Out of nowhere, a yellow jacket stung me on the side of my neck. It was painful and took a while for me to understand I'd been stung. It was sudden and fast.

Grateful and relieved I had no immediate severe reaction, I continued to walk, drove home, took some antihistamine, and iced the sore area. It was a tangible, vivid example how to stay steady, calm, not panicking when encountering an unpleasant situation — a stingy, unpredicted situation.

Funny enough, that whole weekend was comprised of encountering and bumping into similar situations that were uncalled for, unpleasant, and (obviously) out of my control.

Just by being out there we expose ourselves to both sweet and stingy encounters. While hiding in the corner is not a feasible option, the question is how we handle it.

First, accepting the idea that pain, soreness, and stickiness are all parts of being alive and awake is a good start. By accepting it, we cease our constant tendency to run away from the pain and look for comfort and an instant fix. Sometimes we need to learn the pain and get to know its nature.

When not instantly rushing to avoid or to soothe, we can estimate the situation better and find how to best respond.

In some situations, we realize it's simply a dead end. It may feel like unfinished business, pleading for us to continue trying to improve or change it. The sour taste feels prominent and far from joyous. But as painful as it is, with courage we can halt an already sinking motion and avoid dragging ourselves deeper with it.

With that new perception and understanding of the situation, we can look into the pain, stand side by side with it, and still avoid pursuing action on our end. In these circumstances, our further actions are pointless, not bringing different results or anything to fruition.

Living with the loss is difficult. Many times it goes against the grain, but sometimes it's the smarter way. It's not always the case, but sometimes it is, and we need to confront it. It's much wiser to direct our efforts elsewhere.

Like an elite skater, ballet dancer, or actor who knows when to retire: at the top. There's a great deal of loss when it happens on their end. But there's a path to admiration, respect, and appreciation, for good.

Everything is impermanent. We must cease struggling against the reality of drastic and uncontrollable change and instead work with it. When we drop our propensity to cling to the reality we want, we're more capable of working with the reality we have. When we free ourselves of grasping to our internal stories, we're free to spend our energies in a positive direction instead of burying ourselves in a miserable numbing trap, a trap with no light showing us the way to escape.

Challenging times, more than ever, are when we need to practice connecting with the present moment. Connecting with the present moments allows us to take a pause even as we're stuck in the whirlwind. We slow down. We allow ourselves to sit vulnerable, afraid, without pretensions, prejudices, or pre-judgements that blind us and limit our ability to find the answers. We try to come back to the present through our breath.

Again and again, we return to the breath, allowing hundreds of thoughts to come up and to dissipate. We cultivate resilience, sitting with discomfort.

Gentle Reminder

Most worthwhile endeavors require hard work and working through discomfort and challenges. By accepting that we need to work with and through uncomfortable situations, we gain the strength to do so and to achieve more. We can flow with the discomfort and hardship rather than resisting it and find the most effective way forward.

CHAPTER 22:
Slack Water and the Doldrums

We're frequently caught in between. We're waiting for an answer or a package, having no control. We're frequently stuck in holding patterns, waiting for the other shoe to drop.

Slack water. The tides stand still. Between the tides, the water is motionless, giving no hint of the rapid changes that will occur when the time comes.

Floating in slack water resembles being stuck in the doldrums. Like a sailing ship trying to cross the equator, the winds die, the sails fall slack, and the sailors would be forced to tide over (float with the tide). One can only imagine the tremendous frustration those sailors felt as the winds died and the water stood motionless. It must have been long, tedious, and scary. Stuck in position, waiting for the tide to move them, or better yet for a sign of even the lightest breeze that signals freedom from a seemingly endless holding pattern. Weeks can pass in the heat without the slightest hint of progress.

In the Midst

The COVID years made all of us feel like old-time sailors stuck in doldrums. We were stuck in a holding pattern, confined to our ship with no signs of progress. The slack water and air created a vacuum of painful stillness. As we sat, there were signs that the breeze might pick up and the tide would begin to flow in the right direction.

Vaccines arrived. The weather improved. Schools came back, offering more and more in-person learning. The world showed signs of opening up again. Staples of our past lives began to appear again. Places where the majority of people had been vaccinated returned to "normal" and allowed us a glimpse of what was upcoming.

Still, in 2021, we weren't there . . . yet. Instead, we were stuck in a confusing phase where even all the positive signs and optimism were still mired in a dangerous pandemic. We received mixed messages, both uplifting and discouraging.

Even with all the signs, we weren't moving fast enough to feel the progress. The distant point of normality didn't seem to be getting any closer. Nonetheless, inevitably, the tidal stream reversed and helped carry us back to normalcy.

Use the Present

The difficult feeling of being stuck in the doldrums isn't exclusive to the pandemic. It's a common feature of life that we all must face from time to time. We frequently find ourselves waiting and even dependent on actions of others that are completely out of our control. We must cope with the sense of helplessness as we understand we have no ability to control or influence many events that affect our lives intimately or deeply. We're subject to the whims of the weather, waiting for power to come on after a blackout, waiting for a response regarding a proposal we've made, waiting for answers of whether we've been accepted to a college or a new job, or even waiting for package that could arrive any day now. We can be trapped in the doldrums without warning at any time.

When we're stuck in slack water, we can take this time as an opportunity to prepare ourselves. Similar to an airplane that's delayed before takeoff, we have the time to put everything in order.

We warm up our engines. We can check all the equipment to ensure it's working properly. We can position ourselves, facing the direction from where the wind will come. Instead of sinking in frustration and despair, we focus our energy on preparing for our future.

It's a win-win situation. We focus ourselves on creation and doing. We ignite a positive cycle that promotes well-being and a better state of mind. We use the present to cultivate the future we aspire to. We execute now and will reap the benefits sooner than we may imagine.

Gentle Reminder

The times we have in between are an opportunity to prepare. The extra time enables us to stand back and prepare ourselves both emotionally and functionally to be ready for whatever answers or outcomes we must face.

CHAPTER 23:
Dare to Ask

Day-to-day life can overwhelm us. We can fall into ruts just trying to survive. Even as the world constantly changes around us and tries us, we can still access our freedom to choose how we act.

You take a moment to pause.

Stepping back from your life, as if to push the pause button on a remote and put the movie you're watching on hold, the picture stays still. This isn't the typical pause, freezing the movie so you can take a break or get some popcorn without missing any of the action. In this case, it's a different story. The pause is the story. The pause itself has meaning and a purpose. The pause creates an empty space with its own narrative, a story that begins with a void, with room, with no need to add anything. Emptiness is the story.

Entropy begins to take hold. Energy flows to the emptiness. The empty, exposed vessel created by your pause absorbs the heat, light, and sounds that surround it. Staying still, the surrounding energy enters the void, swirling and mixing together. There is a new synergy, a new life, a new creation.

You're tossing a pebble into that void. Causing a ripple, a soundwave that leads to an energetic shift. Potentially, it can upset the pause, breaking it. The strength of the disturbance depends on the angle you're aiming, the amount of strength you use, the speed and size of the thrown pebble.

In all that emptiness, you're daring to ask. What is it that I really want? You toss that pebble courageously without knowing the outcome. Despite the uncertainty, you dare to ask and face the answers that will arise, like sound echoing into the void.

"All that we are is the result of what we have thought. The mind is everything. What we think we become," so said the Buddha.

Unwittingly we can put our life on autopilot. With so much to do and so much responsibility, we stop thinking about what we're doing and why we're doing it. We can become bound to automatic patterns, dragged unthinkingly along by familiar routines, habits, and fears.

We can feel miserable, haunted by the lack of something in our lives. We feel the deficit in the back of our subconscious without knowing or acknowledging it cognitively. Our frustrations can cause us to lash out — blaming certain people, blaming lack of balance, looking for a reason for our frustration. We feel trapped. We, however, are trapped first and foremost by our own minds. Fortunately, our basic nature is to seek freedom. We're driven by instinct to find the path to freedom.

Surprisingly, the answers to the seemingly simple question, "What is it I really want?" aren't easy to find. We assume we know.

When we genuinely pause and search, dare to ask, we find that the picture is a bit more complicated.

Often, we discover we've arrived at a destination for a reason. Despite the assumption that we've been forced into where we are by circumstance, we learn that we may have chosen our path for deeper reasons than we initially suspect.

Taking the time to pause and examine our lives enables us to elevate many issues, new and old, to the surface. Freshly exposed, we can shed a light on them. We develop a new understanding. The people and activities that bring us joy and balance come into focus. We can make the connection of what and who bring joy to our daily lives.

Anything we do in the present impacts the future. It's the law of karma. The simple act of tossing the pebble causes a shift to happen. The way we direct our energy impacts actual outcomes. Asking questions is a form of extending energy outward. By extending energy with our questions, we attract answers and translate those answers into actual changes in our lives.

Our future becomes dough that we can knead. The path we take is not determined by an external power outside of our control, but by the result of our thoughts, purposeful actions, and how we direct our energy. We can always try. We can control our journey.

Gentle Reminder

The ability to pause and take space to see how we arrived where we are now can help us better understand ourselves and better plot our journey forward.

Chapter 24:
A Wake-Up Call for Love

How we act toward others reflects on ourselves. How other people behave toward us is beyond our control. It reveals who they are, not on who we are.

Many years ago in high school, I had the privilege to perform on Israeli TV as part of a youth ensemble. Several members of the ensemble became successful actors and singers and are still performing to this day. Not I. Personally, I left the acting world behind when I was drafted into the air force and never looked back.

Years passed. While I was a member in the ensemble for just two of my teen years, it was an excellent school and is one small part of who I am today.

I was asked to participate in an official reunion for the ensemble. As with many things since the age of COVID-19, the reunion was held via a Zoom video call. The lady who organized it all did a fabulous job. She was able to track down many of the former members of the ensemble. While I never met her in person, I was deeply impressed by her determination. After all, she found me even after all those years and thousands of miles separating me from Israel.

For me, it was pure joy to see and talk with friends I hadn't seen in thirty years. We used to be very close, and at the time we all had a wonderful relationship with no backbiting or drama. The reunion included people from many "generations" of the ensemble, most of whom I didn't know. Still, it was worth the time and effort to see and speak with my old friends.

The artistic director of the ensemble is an extremely talented person (some people claim he's a genius) but a person with a "difficult" personality. Back in the day, I had the personal displeasure of experiencing his "difficult" personality. He often inflicted emotional damage strong enough to feel as if it were a physical assault. As unpleasant as it was at the time, it didn't leave me with any emotional scars or have any deep impact. I simply moved on to better things. Despite this, I can appreciate his abilities, charisma, and charm. I am not a bit surprised that his career and reputation have only grown as the years passed.

A few hours after the Zoom call, a member was sharing a long text he received from the director who didn't participate in the video conference. The reunion had been streamed on Facebook, and he heard some of the comments made about the experience of working under him.

The text was nasty, insulting, deliberately hurtful, and completely unproductive. The intent of the text seemed to be hurtful and to denigrate specific people. Personally, I was untouched; I was not a victim, but it did hurt many others. It was so unnecessary. It stank so bad, even I experienced the odor from thousands of miles away.

I strongly felt the injustice. I try to live and breathe the values of yoga and meditation. The text violated the principle of *ahimsa*, the first yama (see "Chapter 20: Answering Aggression" on page 103 for a deeper dive into the yamas). *Ahimsa* calls for not causing harm in actions, in words, intentions, or thoughts. Not causing harm to ourselves. Not causing harm to others.

We have free will. Everything we do is our choice, and therefore we're responsible for everything we do and say. Everything we do matters. It really does. Given the fact that we are all fallible mortals that have moments of weakness and anger, we bear the burden of moderating our own reactions. Our reactions and responses are entirely our own responsibility. Almost invariably we're forced to cope in the present time. We rarely have the luxury of being able to withdraw, consult with advisors, and make a wise decision. Even in these rare cases, we still need to be able to set aside our own emotions and ego and accept wise advice. We need to be kind to ourselves and others because we all have our difficult moments. I encourage each one of us to slow down and check in with ourselves before acting or speaking. It's a free way to improve our quality of life, our joy, our friendships, and our well-being. Regardless of our motives and intentions, we all cause harm. We can, however, acknowledge it, understand how it happened, and mitigate the harm we cause others.

We have the freedom to avoid poisoning the water in the well we all share. The text was a wake-up call for love and to remind us to pursue the practice of *ahimsa*. May we love ourselves, may we love others, may we all be loved.

Gentle Reminder

We can choose our behavior and the atmosphere we create around ourselves. By pursuing the path of non-harm toward ourselves and others, we are helping ourselves and ensuring that our lives are better.

Chapter 25:
Aging Ouch

We are caught in between the desire to stay young, healthy, and vital forever and the reality that aging, in the end, cannot be stopped.

Technology gets better and better. A vaccine was produced in under a year — a process that usually takes a few years if not more. A rover landed on Mars. Artificial intelligence is beginning to become a reality that we work with every day. Electric cars have gone from a curiosity to a standard part of day-to-day life.

In so many areas, we now have so much knowledge along with the ability to shape it into tangible tools. Going forward the innovative route continues, bringing more and more solutions and products. Just watching a movie from the 90s, we can't help but smile when seeing the character's cell phone. A dinosaur of a flip phone even compared to a first-generation smartphone.

Generally speaking, life expectancy grows, and its quality — at least in potential — as well. Fifty is the new thirty, some say. Sixty is the new forty.

Proper lifestyle, including exercise, diet, and self-care all make a big difference. We have a choice how to conduct our lives, and we are so lucky.

Impermanence is a key element in Buddhism. Everything changes all the time. We can accept this or resist it. We can choose to ignore reality by working against it, trying to form our own reality, or simply work with it. In some cases, our own initiative and energy can form something new — to some degree. Depending on the subject matter, it can become the beginning of a new entity like an entrepreneur starting a company from scratch. It causes a new chain reaction and energy resulting in a smooth addition to the universal experience. Now many of these once-novel ideas like electric cars and artificial intelligence are simply part of our lives.

The challenge is in the situations where our humble abilities are limited . . . limited when meeting the mountain of reality. Reality is still there and not bothering our emotional state. Our minds can be our friend or our worst enemy. How do we manage the frustration and tension between our capabilities and ambitions?

We wake up in the morning, wash our face, and a new line is showing. It doesn't go anywhere. We're aging. Gravity has its impact, no matter if we practice inversions. Our skin might be wonderful thanks to our decent lifestyle, but we age. We think out loud how to best apply the wonderful new anti-aging technology, if at all.

In many interviews celebrities will express their legitimate answer to dermatologist interventions: every person should follow what's right for them. Of course. It's a personal choice that needs to address one's needs, priorities, and happiness.

With that, I suggest that the root for finding contentment is deeper. Whether deciding to avoid interventions or go with them, we may all fall to the vicious cycle of never-ending lack of satisfaction. Its toxicity causes us so much misery. No matter the route we choose. To break that negative cycle, we can find self-acceptance.

As Pema Chödrön reminds us, the key to self-acceptance is that the more connected you are with the unchanging

Self, the less you suffer from the inevitable changes of the non-Self.

Towards the end of a *yoga nidra* guided meditation, we reach the unconditional place within, one of pure awareness, a free zone. It's solid and feels like an internal stone we can stand upon. It gives us an option to widen our narrow perception and story, to allow more self-love.

> Yoga nidra is an ancient practice that consists of a guided meditative journey. Practice lying down with the goal of including full-body relaxation and a deep meditative state of consciousness.

Gentle Reminder

Denying reality will not change it. By taking a pause, we can appreciate ourselves and our strengths, and we can better live with change and impermanence.

CHAPTER 26:
Witnessing Pain, a Fresh Take

We must face the reality that relationships aren't always forever. Friendships and relationships can end. The end of any relationship hurts and can feel like a loss with the heavy weight it carries.

Toward the end of a yoga nidra workshop, participants are asked to find their internal witness. There, they observe themselves and their environment from a place that is pure and free from their habitual storylines and attachments.

They view the world as if they are floating on a cloud and cultivate a new perception free from distractions and distortions. They see matters just as they are. With no additions, editorials, or biases.

By standing aside and seeing ourselves and our lives as neutral witnesses, we learn to discern what situations and events act as a primal resource that triggers sharp and instinctive emotional reactions. We realize that our initial responses to situations are a function of who we are.

We understand that our instinctive reaction to a specific situation will trigger a habitual pattern of behavior that we repeat without any thought to whether our habitual patterns are the best answer to the given situation.

Here, learning to act as a witness, we learn a new path. We can find ways to pause, analyze, explore, and respond differently.

As humans, we have the tendency to avoid pain, both physical and emotional. Pain, however, is an inevitable part of our existence. When you encounter a painful situation, ask yourself, "What's my instinctive response?"

Recently, in my own personal experience, I found that I was able to generate a productive response to a painful situation by utilizing my internal witness. In the short term, it's unlikely to take away the pain.

By stepping aside and viewing the situation as it was, I was able to choose the proper path and find the best way forward.

When connecting with others and building personal relationships, we aspire to have life-long friendships. There are times when our aspirations simply aren't realistic. The pain of letting go of a relationship, of losing a friend, can feel like losing a loved one. As a result, we can refuse to accept that the relationship has come to an end. We run back to it again and again trying to clear ourselves of the incessant feeling of unfinished business.

However, from the clear vision of the witness, we understand that our drive to find the perfect resolution is pointless. As painful as it is, we can see that despite our genuine desire for reality to be different, the truth of the situation is unyielding. Any action to sugarcoat or ignore the situation won't bring us the happy outcome we hope for.

The ability to create space around us and view the world as a dispassionate, unbiased witness enables us to see the unvarnished truth. It leaves us with a deeper understanding of our reality that in the long run will enable us to manage the pain and make the best choices possible. It's better to spend our energy on creating a new positive path in our lives than be destined to repeat the same mistakes in an unending cycle of habitual responses.

It takes courage to live with the fact that we all must live with unfinished business.

Gentle Reminder

The ability to act as a witness, to take space, step aside, and see the truth may seem harsh, but it actually protects us. It enables us to accept reality and can prevent us from harming ourselves pursuing relationships that have already ended or hurt us.

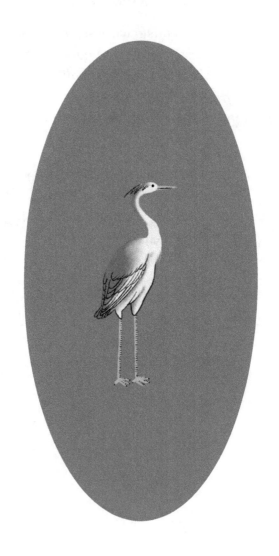

1 It's our decision how we react to aggression and whether we want to add fuel to the fire or, alternatively, find creative ways to reduce it.

2 Living with loss is very difficult. It goes against our natural instincts, but many times it's the smarter way forward. We must be willing to understand the reality of a situation — if it's irreversible or irreconcilable. In that case, it's much wiser to direct our efforts toward something new.

3 When we drop our propensity to cling to the reality we want, we're more capable of working with the reality we have. When we free ourselves of clinging to our internal stories, we're free to spend our energies in a positive direction instead of burying ourselves into a miserable, numbing trap with no light showing us the way to escape.

4 Stuck as we are, we can take this time as an opportunity to prepare ourselves. Instead of sinking in frustration and despair, we can focus our energy on planning for our future. We use the present to cultivate the future we aspire to have.

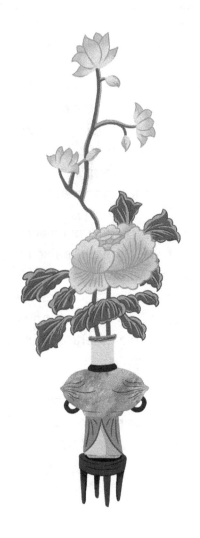

SECTION 4:

REALITY

We choose how we approach reality. What's the proper balance between accepting reality as it is and attempting to change it? In either case, acceptance is the first step. It's the baseline for making a decision and moving forward. When we face reality in the starkest terms possible rather than ignoring or suppressing them, we make the best decision regarding whether simply to move forward with acceptance or take the initiative and attempt to change reality. To find the proper balance in any given situation, only by confronting reality as it truly is can we start with a fresh, open mind and intelligently decide on the best course of conduct.

Our attitude makes the difference. A positive approach can help us whether we are trying to accept a situation or trying to change it. A positive approach creates positive energy that penetrates everywhere, accumulates power, and develops its own momentum. The alternative — sticking our heads in the sand and denying reality — doesn't afford us with the ability to change reality or even to manage it properly.

CHAPTER 27:
A Bump in the Road

There's the famous saying that the weakest link defines the strength of a chain. Like a chain, when it comes to our personal journey, it's important not to let one individual event or challenge break the chain and derail the journey.

Imagine yourself walking along a beautiful path in nature. You cross mountains and valleys. You encounter rivers and lakes. Trees and flowers run alongside the trail. At times, the weather is sunny, at times rainy, at times tranquil, and at times stormy. The path is long, very long. The view from above at a distance is idyllic, but the reality seen up close can be very different.

Nothing goes perfectly to plan. Even as we move smoothly, there always seems to be one item that gums up the works and stops us in our path. We need to be able to keep our momentum and not allow obstacles to knock us off track.

In nature, as we know from our personal experience, even the most beautiful path is far from perfect. In nature, there are no straight lines and few smooth surfaces. Nature is filled with obstacles and annoyances. There are rocks, ditches, and roots to trip over, insects, thorns, and other unexpected, hidden impediments.

You never know when you'll hit a bump in the road. It's easy to acknowledge that our world is strewn with all sorts of obstacles. It's not a source of pain to admit we rarely get the opportunity to travel over a perfectly manicured route.

As in nature, our own personal way is complex and filled with uncertainty and unforeseen challenges. The bumps and divots we encounter on our personal journey can sabotage our way forward, defining the road ahead independent of our will and vision. The question is, do we have the ability to transcend above the obstacles we find in our way? Can we acknowledge when we've hit a bump? Do we have an effective coping mechanism to prevent ourselves from falling from the trail? Many times, we find ourselves falling into a trap because we forget or fail to see that the path is wider than the obstacle. Simply put, we need the wisdom to see that the bump in the road isn't an insurmountable challenge that prevents us from moving forward in the right direction.

We want to cultivate the ability to acknowledge the bump without spiraling into negative actions and reactions. We have the power to choose whether our mind and thoughts are an ally or a burden. We have two options. The first is to turn the bump into something a bit more neutral. We don't pretend that everything is great, but we have the gumption to acknowledge reality and continue to move forward. The second is to refuse to recognize the bump, trip over it, and let it determine our way forward. After stumbling, we get up, dust ourselves off, and continue moving with a clear mind to determine the best way forward. The more we travel and encounter bumps in the road, the more we learn how to recover and more importantly, how to identify bumps in the road before we stumble over them. The more we travel, the more we learn, the more trust we have in our abilities.

As humans, we have been gifted the power of freedom of choice. We all fall. The question is: do we rise up? That's our choice.

Gentle Reminder

When we hit obstacles in our path, we need to be able make space and understand our situation. By making space we can objectively analyze what we're facing and make the proper decision going forward. We can avoid spiraling into an abyss of frustration.

CHAPTER 28:
About Perfectionism

We want to be perfect, to be able to complete any task or win any competition without a blemish. Mistakes are inevitable, and we must work with the understanding that the idea is to do our job as well as possible, not to be perfect.

In *When Things Fall Apart*, Pema Chödrön compares perfection to death (Chödrön 1996).

"Perfection is like death. It doesn't have any fresh air. There is no room for something to come in and interrupt all that. We are killing the moment by controlling our experience."

She explains that by insisting on perfection, we set ourselves up for failure. Eventually, sooner rather than later, we will confront an experience we can't control. Perfectionism is an aggressive approach to life, as we reject experiences whenever they aren't perfect or pleasant. To be fully alive and awake, we need to experience every moment, "perfect" or not.

Wow.

I was raised to be a perfectionist. My genius father was a perfectionist when it came to teaching me proper Hebrew. It was a great tool. I owe him my sparkling clean grammar and expressions to this day. When it came to other areas, things were a bit more rigid for me: ballet dancing for years since I was three, years of piano lessons, becoming the best student in school, the best athlete.

The world was very clear — black and white. Second place felt like a failure.

My mother was not a perfectionist. She always told me a B was enough.

Only now do I realize how brilliant she was in her approach. She was a very successful, professional, and diligent worker, but she was soft enough to stay grounded. Obviously, things got more complicated as I grew up. The youngest of three, I followed two much older brothers who were revered and admired . . . while I was left behind. To me, it felt as if the family revolved around my beautiful, successful, smart, popular, and sought-after brothers. I think my father admired them.

No matter what I did, it felt irrelevant and unimportant. I won a part performing on TV with a teen group — nothing to write home about. Later serving in the Israeli Air Force, when I got an award of excellence, it was no special occasion. When I was best, it was no big deal. When I wasn't, I had no real tools to avoid drowning in emotional turmoil.

A Bit about Figure Skating

March 2015, 2 am

My husband and I are wildly awake and shaking, eyes glued to a laptop between us. I know I need to teach a morning class the next day. I'll be exhausted. It may be crazy, but knowing I had to get up early no matter what is reassuring. Knowing no matter the result, life will go on.

My daughter is about to start her short program at the ISU World Figure Skating Championships in Shanghai, China.

The girl isn't even seventeen years old. It's her second world championship. The previous year, she went to "Worlds" in Tokyo, ready seemingly out of nowhere. She earned her qualifying scores to compete, so she did. Super talented, she's always been a wild card.

Shanghai's a different game. She has trained for almost a year with the most renowned coaches in the world. She's been living in Toronto by herself with a foster family, without her parents there. Her peers are Olympic and World medalists (even gold). They're the best of the best skaters in the world. In training she's shown she has the talent to compete at that level. She's a mesmerizing artist and skater to watch — huge triple jumps, gorgeous lines, and heart-melting movements. She has the whole package, and she and her coaches have expectations.

We're watching the live stream in bed with the familiar feeling of nausea creeping up on us. My husband is now out of bed pacing across the room like a restless tiger. Suddenly, she's on. Looking amazing, she's so pretty with her hair tied back in a perfect ponytail. The TV cameras love her delicate, angular facial features. A smooth, black, sparkly unitard hugs her lean body. A packed arena, her federation, and the judges all have their eyes on her as she takes the ice. Many more eyes watching her on the live broadcast.

She begins. The short program in figure skating is the gateway to the free skate (the finals). If you make more than one mistake, you're done. Years of training boils down to three unforgiving minutes.

In the senior short, there are no double jumps allowed. We knew her tendencies; we knew the programs by heart.

We knew she was a perfectionist. We knew she was afraid to fall.

She starts well, flowing and at ease. Then comes the first jump. We are holding our fingers, breath, and every muscle in our bodies. She pops it. Ugh, only two rotations. Then the second, a triple-triple combination.

She completes a double-triple and loses more vital points.

That's it, done. She didn't fall. It was beautiful skating. "Perfect." But the gate to the free skate and an invitation to the Senior Grand Prix is closed. If on her first jump she'd attempted a triple and fallen, she would've made the free skate, but she popped, lost points, and fell short by the smallest margin.

We wait for her telephone call right after, crying, miserable. We've been there so many times before. Through the many victories and disappointments, we've experienced it all. Looking backward, it was the curse of perfectionism, the fear of falling that held her back.

Gentle Reminder

The pursuit of perfection is paralyzing. Accepting that mistakes will be made doesn't mean accepting subpar performance or not trying to learn from our mistakes, so we can improve. If we're focused on perfection, it will prevent us from taking any action for fear of making a mistake.

CHAPTER 29:
A Beginner's Mind

Experience can be both a teacher and a straitjacket. We need to be able to access the wisdom of our experience without it limiting our ability to see the world in a fresh light and generate new ideas and innovations.

One of my students, an accomplished equestrian, was sharing her experiences from a recent competition. The horse she'd ridden for many years had retired from jumping, and she'd been jumping for a few months on a new horse, a young one. She was telling us how fascinating it was to experience the joy, courage, and trust that the young horse had. Unfettered by bad experiences, the horse could approach each new experience free from fear and anxiety. The horse had a beginner's mind.

When practicing *asana* yoga, we have an opportunity to choose a beginner's mindset. We can, through our intention, determine how we experience our practice. When we're faced with a familiar yoga pose, we stay open to exploring the impact of the pose with no assumptions. Each time we practice a pose, we have a unique independent experience. Each day, we can feel something new.

We avoid operating on autopilot by exploring how we enter and how we exit each pose. We can study the rhythm of our breath, the awareness of when we hold it. We can focus on a different part of our body each time we practice a pose to receive a new perception.

Changing the physical reality can help evoke the beginner's mind. We can use props to reframe our body in the pose, practice next to a wall, or use a barre. Sometimes circumstances can change our reality; practicing with an injury can force us to have a new experience when attempting common poses.

Students find the ability to harness the beginner's mind keeps their practice fresh and helps them avoid falling into a rut.

Practicing without a beginner's mindset can lure us into habitual patterns composed solely of muscle memory. We can unconsciously repeat misalignments and fall into previous patterns. The lack of awareness makes us vulnerable to repeating damaging habits that risk our safety and sabotage our ability to extract the best experience out of our practice.

Accumulating experience does have its advantages. As we practice, we learn. We accumulate positive experiences that bring us back to the mat again and again. The positive experiences we feel while practicing yoga are instilled in our body, breath, and mind. This shift we feel is the result of the routine called *asana* yoga. The more we repeat it, the more we can deepen it, and the self-journey is endless. We become effective, and because of our familiarity with the process we can divert our gaze to new points or areas to focus on.

Where is the balance between building on our experiences and keeping a beginner's mind? How do we build on our experience and accumulated wisdom with a beginner's mind? A beginner's mind is like an internal guard that reminds us to stay open to whatever arises. A beginner's mind can break out of the rigid structures created by our experience. It helps us extend beyond past experiences to make new discoveries and learn more about ourselves and our practice.

Off the mat in our daily lives, being trapped by our previous experiences manifests itself in how it can limit our perception and our ability to see the world in its entirety. Depending solely on previous experiences colors our new experiences and present encounters. It masks our senses and blocks our ability to sincerely learn, grow, and change.

It's true that relying on our experience helps us cope by using accumulated wisdom to try to predict the outcome of familiar events, but looking at the world through narrow lenses won't help us cope with new and novel situations. It may blind us to the world around us.

A beginner's mind enables us to maintain a natural flow that helps us manage the impermanence and constant evolution found in nature. Everything is constantly changing, sometimes slower and sometimes faster. Regardless of the pace of change, change is a phenomenon we need to accept and work with in accordance with a shifting reality.

A beginner's mind is a golden tool for facing our fears. Experience can evoke a set reaction of self-doubt and anxiety. We're all susceptible to moments of weakness. A beginner's mind helps us look beyond fear and self-doubt and build new positive experiences we can use as a catalyst to move forward.

Adopting a beginner's mind when relating to our own pattern of ingrained reactions is a gift. Here, we can choose how to perceive self-doubt. Instead of seeing our fears as an implacable enemy, we can appreciate the wake-up call and remind ourselves not to take anything for granted. We stay awake and open to exploring what we can learn and what new perspective we can take from each experience. We have the courage to learn from it, respect it; we move forward from the experience with a chance to grow and pick a different route in life.

Instead of wearing our experience like a heavy, suffocating mask, we leverage our experience to have a light touch, allowing us to play, explore, and taste each experience to the fullest.

RECOMMENDED PRACTICE

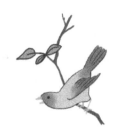

CHOOSE ANY (OR ANY COMBINATION) OF THE SEQUENCES FROM THE "MORNING & NIGHT HOME PRACTICE WORKSHOP" ON PAGE 179. APPROACH THE SEQUENCE WITH A BEGINNER'S MINDSET, SO IT WILL FEEL AS IF IT'S THE FIRST TIME YOU HAVE EVER PRACTICED THE SEQUENCE.

Gentle Reminder

When we're facing a challenge, one of the most effective ways of finding a solution is taking the space needed to set aside our preset notions and see the problem from a new angle or a new light. The beginner's mind allows us to find new ways to view and approach problems and to find better solutions that are relevant to the present.

CHAPTER 30:
Going against the Grain

There's a difference between maintaining healthy habits and being stuck on autopilot, operating mindlessly. Making a change in our habitual patterns can create an opportunity to evaluate where we are.

In *viloma pranayama*, a breath technique, students learn to manipulate their habitual pattern of breathing. In this technique, they're guided to split either their inhale or exhale into three distinct parcels. In between each parcel there's a pause when the breath is suspended.

When splitting inhalation, the student inhales for a count and suspends the breath, continues to inhale for an additional count and suspends the breath again, and then takes the final count of the inhale and suspends the breath again.

The split inhalation is followed by a long, deep exhalation of breath. It's a wonderful exercise that deepens the breath, bringing calmness and relaxation. *Viloma*, ironically, is described as "going against the grain."

By changing our unconscious pattern of breath and introducing a new pattern of breath, we create a shift in our body and our mind.

Routine vs. Reality

It was a gorgeous autumn afternoon. The air was crisp, the temperature pleasant, the skies were clear. The conditions could not be better for a walk in fresh air.

For me, a walk in fresh air is my daily pause. It's where I accumulate energy, release excess pressure from my body and mind, and boost my mood. I will take my walk in almost any type of weather.

Even when it's not convenient, I'll usually be able to squeeze it into a hectic schedule between work, family, and household obligations.

Given the benefits and its positive impact on me, I will insist on my walk regardless of my mood, level of exhaustion, or even lack of desire. Overcoming my reluctance and exhaustion has invariably proven to be a smart decision.

That beautiful afternoon, after a particularly intense period of nonstop work, I found myself taking off my sneakers. I was about to leave the house for a walk, but I stopped — going against my grain. I realized that I was moving by force of habit, stuck on a default course.

During the previous few days, I'd felt the signs of physical exhaustion — sore muscles and fatigue. To stay healthy, I had to dial it back. I had to go against my grain, and for once to refrain from the tendency to push myself. My instinct is to do, to take the initiative and never let myself take a day off no matter what. Only by taking a pause and allowing myself to see reality in the starkest terms was I able to understand that this time, I needed to make a change. In this case, I needed to go against the grain.

Going against the grain can open the breath. It can help us take a pause from constant effort to find a path of health and well-being. Going against the grain requires us to keep our hearts and minds genuinely open to the truth. It can be tricky, to cease our tendency to hold onto a fixed set of perceptions and opinions. We have to have the courage to release our hold on comfortable familiar places. We need to dare to tread outside the familiar where it may be unknown and scary. When we go against our own grain, we may release ourselves from old patterns and find a feeling of freedom and release we've never felt before.

We provide our mind its own fresh breath of air, enabling us to expand beyond our boundaries.

Gentle Reminder

It can be healthy to take a break. We tend to be constantly on the go driven by habit, pressure, or the fear of missing out. By occasionally interrupting our usual patterns, even healthy ones, we tune into our needs and promote balance. Taking a well-timed recovery day can help us better evaluate where we are. We recharge, so we can move forward with renewed vigor.

CHAPTER 31:
The Boo-Hoo Token Jar

We accumulate so much in life. We not only amass material possessions, but also emotional baggage that can weigh us down.

The savings jar — a fun and often effective way to simultaneously save money and incentivize self-improvement. Whether it's a jar to remind us to do our chores or a basic "swear jar" to get us to clean up our language, it's a physical embodiment we use to unburden ourselves of bad habits. It's a good idea that we can take to another level.

We can create a new mental jar, one that together with the tools of yoga and meditation, we can use to release ourselves from the hardships and emotional burdens that hold us back and keep us in a rut. It's the boo-hoo token jar. The jar can be any size, shape, or color. Unburdened, we can move forward with our lives a bit wiser and a little freer of the emotional chains that can bind us.

Our lives are so full of experiences and relationships that it's inevitable we encounter challenges and disappointments on an almost daily basis. By recognizing and accepting these hardships, we're able to let them go, move forward, and be kinder and more understanding to ourselves and the people in our lives.

The Source of Tension and Anxiety

Think of a personal relationship that's a source of pain. For example, you envision that your children can be friends and develop relationships with other family members of a similar age. You have a vision of deepening family relationships and creating bonds that bridge borders. Instead, all your efforts are greeted with a cold shoulder.

It's as if you're trying to play catch with a person who refuses to catch the ball, let alone throw it back. Despite years of trying with the most genuine intentions, you can make no headway. Logically, it seems like a simple and easy mission, but the reality is completely different. There's no effort to reciprocate. After years of trying, the whole endeavor turns out to be a dead end. There's now unbearable tension between your hopes and the disappointment of reality. This tension can lead to feelings such as anger, anxiety, and frustration — feelings that can pull us into an emotional tailspin. It happens to all of us, and we are all susceptible to it.

The question is how we cope, grow, and move forward when feeling the effects of the tension of our expectations going unmet. What strategies and tools do we have to enable us to move on with our lives in a positive and meaningful way?

Let Go of Self-Deception

As in meditation practice, you develop the courage to face things as they are in their rawest, most unvarnished form. This confrontation with the plain facts, painful as it may be, compels you to shed layers and feel naked and exposed in front of the ringing truth. Apply that ability here to confront reality. Face the situation, allow yourself to touch the pain. Explore its nature. Adopt a courageous clear view, with no dissembling. This initial step can take time and effort.

Prepare for an uneasy experience. The experience requires us to overcome our natural instinct to avoid pain.

◇◇◇

RECOMMENDED PRACTICE

TRY THE "MEDITATION" ON PAGE 188
TO PRACTICE STAYING STILL, CREATING
THE OPEN SPACE NEEDED TO SEE REALITY
WITHOUT FILTERS.

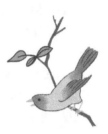

◇◇◇

Congratulations on Your Courage in Facing the Unvarnished Truth

The next step, which carries its own challenge (no one promised it would be a light, airy process), is all about acceptance. The ability to surrender and accept reality isn't a sign of weakness, rather it's a sign of courage, a quality of the "warrior" to be willing to face and accept the truth. It's the ability to understand graciously that sometimes we lose. It's to build the strength needed to admit that in this particular game and on this particular court, we've lost. We must overcome our excuses and desires for an alternate reality to surrender to the present reality. It's the acceptance that we're human, and as humans we're vulnerable and fallible. We all must cope with disappointment and failure. So here we are. Through courage and perseverance, you now have a clear view of reality. You accept it's a waste of energy to repeat previous mistakes. It's time to let go.

Introducing: The Boo-Hoo Token

This token is a representation of your achievements so far. Now that you can clearly recognize reality and accept it, you're able to let it go and move forward. The disappointment has been captured and encapsulated in a token, a boo-hoo token, that can be set aside and left behind in the boo-hoo token jar. Free of this burden, you can now move forward. It addresses your courage and strength not to be a servant to negative feelings, but to have the freedom to make the choice how and where you spend your energy and efforts. You are a warrior. The acceptance of your vulnerability, fallibility, and humanity is a representation of your inner courage and wisdom. You decide is to let go. You drop the boo-hoo token in the jar. You may shed a tear or many tears as you let go. Boo-hoo, but you're free.

Explore a Wonderful New Space

You have an opportunity to pursue new fruitful and beneficial endeavors. Fresh turf may reward your efforts with reciprocity. A new place justifies your energy and emotional investment. Nothing is the promised land. Failures, suffering, and unwanted situations will always be a part of our lives. Being consumed by disappointment is our decision, but it's all within our power to free ourselves of the emotional ties that hold us down. After all, life is too short. We cry, boo-hoo, and then we let go and begin to smile.

Gentle Reminder

Space allows us to acknowledge disappointments and frustrations. Only by recognizing and identifying our emotional challenges can we set them aside and move forward unburdened. We're free to work and react from a clean place.

CHAPTER 32:
Exiting the Tunnel

As our life situations change, we can adapt to vastly different realities. They become the norm. If we live with anxiety, we can get used to living with anxiety, and it becomes routine. When change comes, and the source of the anxiety disappears, we must reacquaint ourselves with a return to what we once considered normalcy. It can be harder than we'd imagine.

A baby was born in the beginning of the COVID-19 pandemic. At the time, none of us could imagine the length and depth of the pandemic and how it would affect each of our lives. As the new reality became clear, the responsible parents formed a safe social pod and didn't allow exposure to the baby besides her sister and themselves. For a while, her relatives were only able to watch the beautiful girl develop from afar or through a windowpane. Over time, as the need to social distance lessened, the baby was introduced to the remainder of her family. She experienced the chaos and noise of cousins for the first time after months of relative isolation and quiet.

Even for an outgoing and developed baby, this new experience, all the stimulation, was a bit overwhelming. She had advanced cognitive skills for her age, but even for her, this new experience was a little too overpowering. What was once a normal experience that almost every baby grows up with had become something novel, something entirely new.

A preschool teacher shared with us her experience of having her group of preschoolers draw a face. Before COVID-19, many children that age would forget to draw the nose. This year, they forgot to draw a mouth. When the teacher asked the students what they forgot in their drawing of a face, the universal answer was, "Oh, we forgot our masks!"

COVID-19 upended our natural habitual patterns. Before, most people sought social interaction and would gravitate towards a crowd. Being packed into a space with people was normal and, in most cases, even desirable. During the pandemic, however, normal human behavior and instincts became dangerous. People are social animals who seek safety in numbers and community, an instinct that became a peril amid an airborne virus. It was potentially a matter of life and death. People adapted quickly to the new reality and learned how to stay safe. This new reality created a new set of habits and instincts that are not so easy to shake. Our COVID-19 protection mechanism has become an ingrained habit.

Once we saw the light at the end of the tunnel, we climbed out of the pandemic. Surprisingly, the fresh rays of the sun we prayed for brought a mixed bag of emotions.

From the many conversations I've had, whether in meditation sessions, at the studio, or even at school, the thought of returning to a pre-COVID world without restrictions was a source of anxiety. For example, many people worried they lost their social skills, which they fear diminished over time unused. In addition, the speed of the change from lockdown to almost completely unrestricted caught many people by surprise. There was little time to adapt to the shift in our reality. We were overwhelmed when forced out of our cocoons. We were still trapped in our survival mode but were compelled to no longer view human contact as inherently dangerous.

Impermanence is at the core of Buddhist beliefs. Our breath comes and goes, an inhale is followed by an exhale, and that exhale is followed by the next inhale and so forth. Our thoughts rise and evaporate, just like the breath. When meditating we learn to notice thoughts. Fears and stories are not as solid or as implacable as they may seem. Nothing is. Just as impermanence applies to our thoughts and lives it also applies to the COVID-19 pandemic. It happened and has slowly morphed out of a part of normal life, just like a long exhale.

How Do We Manage Abrupt Change?

To begin with, let's accept it. With a gentle approach towards ourselves, let's accept our confusion and difficulty. Simply by learning to relax, without changing anything, we will have put ourselves in a much better position to adapt to a new reality. Relaxation by itself creates the conditions needed to move out of the shadows of our fear. We can apply the skills we've developed in our yoga practice, particularly from yin and restorative yoga, that enable us to stay relatively still regardless of what comes up. We avoid reacting, but we notice our initial thoughts and learn from them. We stay still with patience and calm, knowing that the merry-go-round will turn, and we can catch it by waiting for it to come back around instead of desperately chasing it in circles.

In place of fixed judgements and prejudices, we can maintain an attitude of openness and curiosity toward the new age and whatever it brings. Our breath can be an anchor to let us return to the present moment, engaging in the now. Focusing on the here and now gives us the ability to find solid ground to stand upon regardless of the turmoil around us.

Finally, as situations change constantly, we learn how to keep a light approach and maintain our humor, observing the big picture, and not falling into traps of fear or old habits. We can soften our approach to the world, trusting our solid core to keep us stable and strong.

RECOMMENDED PRACTICE

TRY ANY OF THE RESTORATIVE SEQUENCES IN OUR "SUGGESTED NIGHT SEQUENCE FOR HOME PRACTICE" ON PAGE 185 TO CALM THE PARASYMPATHETIC NERVOUS SYSTEM AND FIND RELAXATION.

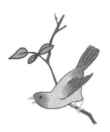

Gentle Reminder

Adapting to a new reality, even a positive change, takes time. We must understand that it's a process that cannot be skipped or shortened. Only by truly acknowledging and identifying change can we take the time and space we need to adapt and move forward in a positive and confident manner relevant to the new present.

Chapter 33:
Decision Making Is Hard

We're faced with decision making on a daily basis. Decision making, even in seemingly trivial situations, can be challenging. We need to be able to make decisions that are not only correct but also that we can live with peacefully.

"Decision making is hard, but when we consider the welfare of others, it becomes very simple."
— Sakyong Mipham Rinpoche

Is it that simple? One of my studio's key values is that "All Are Welcome." Being inclusive to whoever wants to come and practice yoga and meditation with us is core to our mission as a studio that's open to all. For us, differentiating between people for any reason, be it age, gender, politics, race, religion, sexuality, or any other reason, is wrong. As one of our core beliefs, we never thought it could possibly clash with another one of our core beliefs — the safety, health, and well-being of our students.

The COVID-19 pandemic, as it had with so many of our basic assumptions, forced us to reconsider our approach. The science and data are clear and indisputable. The only way out of the pandemic which took so many lives and upended the well-being of so many people was through vaccination. History repeats itself. Vaccination has ended the pain and suffering caused by many diseases — polio, measles, mumps, tetanus, whooping cough, and the list goes on and on — and COVID-19 was no exception.

Despite these facts, getting vaccinated became a matter of politics and not a matter of modern medical science. Many people truly felt as if their personal freedom was at stake. We didn't doubt the sincerity of their beliefs. Taking a stand on the issue of vaccination felt that we'd be abandoning one of our core beliefs — that "All Are Welcome." Mandating vaccination felt wrong because it violated the core principle of inclusivity. Disagreeing with someone over politics didn't give us the right to vilify or exclude. Ignoring reality, however, put the safety of all involved — pregnant women, people with preexisting conditions, and people caring for babies or the elderly — at risk and by extension the people they cared for at risk. Despite all our efforts to try and reconcile the two, we were forced to choose between two core beliefs: inclusivity and the safety of our students.

✄

In the Jewish tradition, the sages have a saying: Saving a life overrides the observance of the Sabbath. It may seem obvious, but observance of the Sabbath is a key principle of traditional Judaism.

Many observant Jews will walk miles in the heat or cold on Saturday to attend services. It's core to their being, but the sages are clear. The health and well-being of a fellow human being is the first priority. According to the Mishnah, saving a life at the expense of one Sabbath will enable the person to observe many more Sabbaths to come (Shabbat Tractate of the Mishnah). With this thought, Sakyong Mipham Rinpoche's words ring true as well, and the decision becomes easy.

The word karma means "action." A decision we make now will create an action that will cause an effect. Whether in the short term or the long term, our action will cause a wave of reactions, subtle or intense. Like a stone we throw in a lake, it will create some movement in the water, a shift, a change in the stream, even if minimal.

Encouraged by the opening quote, we make the safety of others and the health of our community our top priority in our decision-making. Chances are we engage the karmic cycle in a manner that will create a positive impact all around. In the end, it was a matter of conscience, and despite the angst and conflict, we felt it was the only path where we could continue our practice while keeping people safe. Knowing this, we accept the idea or karma and take full responsibility for the outcome.

Even when the decision becomes easy, taking responsibility is always hard.

Gentle Reminder

Decisions need to incorporate both our interests and our values. In the real world, we can't ignore our interests. We must, however, be able to balance our interests and our values. Even if we must sacrifice some of our interests, by being loyal to our key values, we will gain the most both personally and professionally.

CHAPTER 34:
Working from Previous Experiences

We must balance the wisdom we've gained with experience, with the ability to maintain an open mind and defy imprisonment in rigid structures of thought. We need to be able to view new experiences and ideas with an open mind, equally able to acknowledge when our previous experience doesn't apply.

I was stepping out of the house at the crack of dawn to take my morning walk. There, in the front yard, I literally bumped into two fawns. Seeing me, they panicked and began to run in circles, with no direction or purpose. They were so rattled, they couldn't even escape from the perceived threat. Their reaction caught me by surprise.

That entire summer, we were surrounded by deer of all sizes and ages, as they ate our garden and enjoyed the dew on the lawn. Despite our efforts to shoo them away with loud noises and wild gestures, the older and larger bucks had a much more measured reaction. Usually they stopped for a moment, observed us, and then continued to chew the plants leisurely. Only after a concerted effort did they slowly make their way to the fence, where they calmly leapt over it and moved on to the next lawn and garden.

The fawns were instantly terrified by my appearance. I did nothing, my mere presence in the garden triggered instinctive fear and a hysterical reaction. As the fawns mature and gain experience, they'll learn, like their parents, to have a much more measured reaction to humans. They'll get used to our presence and understand how best to react.

We too, like the deer, learn how to cope with our surroundings. We experience a situation, react, and learn from each encounter. Our life is a continuous stretch of encounters and experiences with our environment. As we accumulate experiences, we learn how to hone our reactions to best fit the situation. Encounters that at one time generated fear and extreme reactions may now generate a calm and measured response.

In meditation and yoga practices we encourage adopting a beginner's mind (see "Chapter 29: A Beginner's Mind" on page 145). We encourage the practitioner to stay genuinely open to whatever comes up while discarding any prejudices or preconceived notions. It's a refreshing approach that enables students to experience familiar poses in a novel way. In meditation, a beginner's mind empowers the practitioners to set aside the thoughts that bubble up and to see the world in a new light. The beginner's mind enables us to avoid having our practice become stale and repetitive. It prevents the habit of merely drifting away when meditating and supports us in adhering to the basic tenets of meditation. Bringing our attention back to the breath, it allows us to reap the maximum benefit of our practice.

For humans, our ability to continuously learn from our experiences and constantly improve our reactions to the world around us may be our greatest gift.

Even better, there are many paths through which we can pursue wisdom and hone our reactions to our environment.

No single entity or school of thought has a monopoly on wisdom. Once we find our path, we can follow it and gain the wisdom we need to better interact with our world. As we grow wiser, we can apply our knowledge to all aspects of our lives, whether it's to improve our daily routine or get ahead in our career. The more we apply our newly acquired wisdom to our lives, the more we can improve our ability to cope with our world.

The caveat here is when repetition causes rigidity. We become stuck in a rut, and we decide ahead of time what we see and lose the ability to see the world as it truly is. Instead of curiosity we stick to a framework that makes us feel comfortable. The danger is in constantly seeking out the same framework as a means to feel safe and secure. We feel safe in it, even if it's an illusion. We use it to avoid the fear and uncertainty that comes from the new and the unknown.

It's a tough challenge to improve through repetition without falling into the trap of rigidity. Fortunately, there's a way to avoid the trap. By maintaining a beginner's mind, we keep our curiosity and look for new patterns to learn from. We keep our freedom and don't lock ourselves in our illusionary comfort zone.

While we can't control the world around us, we can control our approach and our mindset. In *Living Beautifully: with Uncertainty and Change*, Pema Chödrön reflects on this (Chödrön 2012).

"Chögyam Trungpa had an image for our tendency to obscure the openness of our being; he called it 'putting makeup on space.' We can aspire to experience the space without the makeup. Staying open and receptive for even a short time starts to interrupt our deep-seated resistance to feeling what we're feeling, to staying present where we are."

The beginner's mind helps create the awareness we need to make a shift. We can learn to discern between when we're retreating into our comfort zone and when we see the world and manage its challenges in a realistic and effective manner. As we already learned, regardless of our efforts, we have no control over the events around us and must adapt and learn to successfully overcome each new crisis.

Gentle Reminder

Taking a pause and making space enables us to understand whether our experience and knowledge can provide the answer or whether we need to take a new line of inquiry and approach the situation with a fresh view that's relevant to the current challenge.

CHAPTER 35:
Making a Change

Frequently we face facts and events which challenge our view of the world. We need to be able to take a sober look at ourselves and our world and be able to change our course. This is never an easy task.

The earth is shaking. External circumstances keep banging on your door. As if the volatile uncertainty brought about by the latest external crisis isn't enough, whether it's the economy, a foreign war, or a pandemic, you discover that your personal and professional lives are just as vulnerable to change brought on by outside forces. You're surprised. A bolt out of the blue, you weren't expecting it.

You realize that despite the temptation to put your head in the sand and hope the storm passes you by, it's better to act and take the initiative. In yoga practice, the concept of surrender is encouraged. To accept the reality of the situation and work within one's limits is deemed the wiser course of action.

Surrender, however, doesn't mean passivity. We don't meekly accept whatever the heavens decree. Surrender means to accept that change in a volatile world is inevitable. Surrender means that you have to be proactive in the face of change rather than standing by passively hoping that everything will turn out for the best on its own. You take the courageous step and decide to embrace the change forced on you by the outside world. You decide that despite the discomfort on multiple levels, you will embrace the change and redirect your life. You understand it involves risk and the unknown. You know that every change has its unintended consequences and collateral damage. Most of them are beyond your control.

Despite this, you accept change. You surrender. There's no point in resisting. As always you tune into your own voice and stay loyal to your true self. A new direction doesn't mean you can't be authentic.

Trying to maintain full stillness in a stormy sea is a recipe for failure. Instead, we learn to flow with the currents and find the best way to navigate our new journey.

Surrendering to change enables us to embrace our new reality and better guide ourselves to the changing currents and tides, better adjusting to new conditions.

And yes, there's risk.

One, two, three, and here you are. You've built a new reality that better fits your new circumstances. A mix of excitement and nervousness flush over you. Your new beginning is here, a change has been made.

The start of a new journey, but a journey you're making with the support of all the wisdom you've gained from your past experiences. While you're facing a new world, you have all the tools you need to move forward.

As you travel over new and unfamiliar terrain, you pull on past experiences to help find your footing. The more you move forward, the more you learn. You feel you're gaining traction with each step.

Meeting the discomfort of the unknown, constantly encountering the frustrations from new obstacles, and all the while finding the satisfaction of making new discoveries is your new lot in life.

It's challenging, but you feel alive, so alive. You feel your senses are sharp again. You're so present and in the moment because you're forced to engage in the immediacy of your experience. You're grateful for it, because, after all, you have purpose and the feeling of self-fulfillment.

With curiosity, with fear, with excitement, and with gratitude, you simply appreciate your new way forward.

Gentle Reminder

Being able to surrender and make a change is not a sign of weakness or a sign that everything we've done is for naught. Acceptance is a sign of strength and wisdom. Driving over a cliff just to prove we're always right will always hurt us more than acknowledging the need to make a change. Being able to make a change is what enables us to grow, get stronger, and move forward with confidence. Knowing when to surrender is a sign of maturity and wisdom.

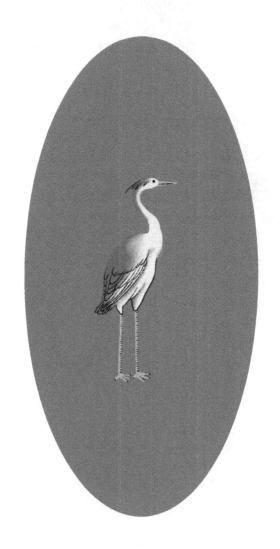

SECTION 4 SIMPLY PUT

1 We have the power to choose whether our mind and thoughts are an ally or a burden. We want to cultivate the ability to acknowledge the bump in the road we face without spiraling into a chain of negative actions and reactions.

2 By insisting on perfection, we prevent ourselves from being fully alive and awake. We need to experience and appreciate every moment whether it's "perfect" or not.

3 By maintaining a beginner's mind, we maintain our curiosity and thereby enable ourselves to learn from new patterns. We keep our freedom and creativity and don't lock ourselves in an illusionary comfort zone.

4 The beginner's mind is able to break out of rigid structures created by our habits and experience. It enables us to see beyond past experiences and to make new discoveries.

5 The ability to surrender and accept reality isn't a sign of weakness, rather it's a sign of courage. It's the quality of the "warrior" to be willing to face and accept the truth. It's the ability to understand graciously that sometimes we fail. The acceptance of your vulnerability, fallibility, and humanity is a representation of your inner courage and wisdom and the starting point for improvement, development, and growth.

WRAP UP &
RESOURCES

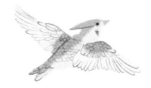

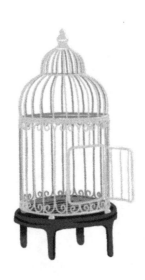

Conclusion

Yoga and meditation go far beyond the boundaries of any studio or class. They can penetrate the very core of any situation or environment. Yoga's core teachings are not just spiritual, they can be practical and useful in our modern world. Through consistent daily practice and thoughtfulness, the ideas and concepts of yoga and meditation offer guidance and insights that enable us to cope with the challenges and hardships that blindside us.

In my life, and in my family members' lives, we have been fortunate enough to overcome our own challenges and hardships by leveraging these lessons. There's practicality beyond the spirituality of yoga. We have found relevance at work, in school, and in our personal relationships. There's no contradiction between striving for success in the material world and striving for personal development. By utilizing the lessons of yoga and meditation, my experience as a career woman and a mother can be mutually beneficial. My experience as a yoga and meditation instructor has shown that students can and frequently do apply these lessons to improve their own lives. Seeing people, family, friends, and students improve their quality of life through ideas taught by yoga and meditation has inspired me in return.

My purpose is to make these lessons and ideas accessible and practical to everyone, whether they're a devout practitioner or a non-yogi. I hope that by offering a window into my life and the lives of the people I love, anyone and everyone can glean lessons that are relevant to their own lives. I hope to offer inspiration and confidence through the truth that the power of these ideas is available to anyone with an open mind. Even a small change and improvement can help you achieve a higher quality of life.

Morning & Night Home Practice Workshop

See h2c.ai/rgx for more resources.

Suggested Morning Sequence for Home Practice

The morning sequence is modular and enables you, the practitioner, to decide to complete the entire sequence or a part of the sequence depending on your needs. Begin with the warm-up (and end there), pick and choose any of the subsequent modules, or complete the whole sequence. In any case, you'll benefit from your practice.

Sitting Warm-Up and Centering

◊ Begin in a comfortable seated position, crossed legs (*sukhasana*) or any other comfortable seated position.

◊ Pause, close your eyes, take a few breaths, pay attention to where you're holding tension in your body.

◊ Reach your hands in prayer in front of your heart center. Reach the hands together in prayer above your head, and release them in a wide arc to the sides of your body. Reverse the motion

(raise them above your head in an arc) and
return to hands in prayer in front of your heart.
Repeat this flow three times.

◊ Reach your hands above your head in prayer,
lean to the right, back to center, and then lean to
the left. Take a twist to the right, placing your left
hand on your right knee for extra leverage, take
a breath, return to center, and then take a twist
to the left, placing your right hand on your left
knee. Take a breath, and return to center.

◊ Extend your hands forward and forward fold.
Take several breaths, and only then slowly and
carefully move to a child pose at the back of
the mat.

Table-Top Warm-Up

◊ Move on your hands and knees — table-
top position.

◊ Tuck your toes under, arch your back (cat),
and inhale.

◊ Untuck your toes, round your spine (cow),
and exhale.

◊ Repeat cat and cow four more times (five times
in total).

◊ After you complete your cat-cow sequence in
table-top position, tuck your toes under, and
straightening your arms and legs, push up into
downward dog.

◊ Hold downward dog for five breaths.

Beginning of Standing Sequence

◊ Walk your legs forward into forward fold at the
front of the mat.

◊ Roll your torso up with a rounded spine, and move to a standing position (*tadasana* or mountain pose) at the front of the mat. Reach your hands in prayer in front of your heart center.

Standing Flow at the Front of the Mat

◊ Reach your hands above your head.
◊ Release your hands to your sides in a wide arc and simultaneously forward fold.
◊ Reach your hands to your shins or thighs and lengthen your spine.
◊ Release into forward fold.
◊ Take a breath and roll up to a standing position.
◊ Repeat the sequence three times.

Lunge Sequence

◊ From a standing position (*tadasana*), take a forward fold, and then extend your right leg back to a lunge.
◊ From your lunge, place your hands on the mat and move back to downward dog by moving your left leg back to join your right leg.
◊ Move from downward dog, rolling your shoulders forward and straightening your back into plank position.
◊ Drop your knees to the mat without lifting your feet.
◊ Release your chest in between your arms while keeping your elbows glued to the side of your body (half *chaturanga*).
◊ Lifting your chest, move to baby cobra and then push back into downward dog.

◊ From downward dog, walk your legs forward to the front of the mat to a forward fold and roll your torso up to a standing position.

◊ Repeat the sequence on the other side, starting the sequence with moving to a lunge by extending your left leg to the back of the mat.

◊ Repeat this flow as many times as your body wants or needs.

Warrior Sequence

◊ Start in a standing pose and forward fold. From a forward fold, move to a lunge by sending your right leg to the back of the mat.

◊ From a lunge, send your left leg back to meet your right and move into downward dog

◊ From downward dog, roll your shoulders forward to a plank pose.

◊ Either hold plank pose, take a half *chaturanga* or, if you're ready, take a full *chaturanga*, lowering your chest past your elbows.

◊ Move back to downward dog.

◊ Send your right leg forward in a lunge, and raise your arms above your head to move to warrior one, exhale and open your chest to the side of the room, arms parallel to your legs in warrior two.

◊ Straighten your front leg, moving to triangle pose. From triangle, release to a lunge, drop your back knee down, raise your arms, and add a back bend. From your back bend, take your hands in prayer and twist to the right. Release your twist and move back to center.

◊ Reach your hands to the floor, lift your back knee, and move and back to downward dog.

◊ Repeat this sequence on your other side by walking your legs forward to a forward fold and rolling up to *tadasana* (standing pose). From a standing pose, forward fold and move to a lunge by sending your left leg to the back of the mat.

◊ Repeat this flow as many times as your body wants or needs.

Balancing Sequence

◊ Walk from downward dog to a standing position at the front of the mat. From a standing position, reach your left knee up and open it to the side, moving to tree pose standing on your right leg.

◊ You may take your hands in prayer in front of your heart center, if you are feeling safe, you may reach your hands above your head and open them away. When you feel you've had enough, reach your hands in prayer (if they're not already there), release your left leg and move back to *tadasana* (standing pose).

◊ Repeat tree pose, standing on your left leg and raising your right knee, repeating the pose as before.

Moving to Rest on Your Belly

◊ From a standing position take a forward fold and extend your right leg back to a lunge. Move back to downward dog by moving your left leg to the back of the mat to meet your right leg.

◊ From downward dog, move forward to plank, drop your knees, and move to lie on your belly.

◊ Take a few moments to rest.

Backbends

- When you're ready, interlace your hands behind your lower back and lift your shoulders, chest, and legs up to a locust pose.
- Hold locust pose for several breaths. When done, release to lie on your belly again.
- Release to a child pose at the back of the mat.

Inversion

- Meet in downward dog.
- If you want, release your forearms down and move into a forearm downward dog.
- Release from forearm downward dog to a child pose.

Bridge Pose

- Move from child pose carefully back to a comfortable seated position.
- Straighten both legs forward and forward fold (*paschimottanasana*).
- Bend your knees, place your feet on the ground, and slowly roll onto your back.
- When you're ready, lift your pelvis up into a bridge pose. Hold the pose for several breaths.

Move to Lie on Your Back

- Release your pelvis to the mat and hug your knees to your chest.
- Drop both knees to the right side in a twist and hold the twist for several breaths.
- Carefully move both legs back to the center, and then twist to the left side.

◊ Return to center. Straighten your legs up to the ceiling. Either stay with your legs up or carefully move into a shoulder stand.

◊ Gently roll down one vertebra at a time to lie on your back and rest in *savasana* for as long as necessary or comfortable.

◊ Move slowly and carefully from *savasana* back to a comfortable seated position. Take several breaths and begin your day.

Suggested Night Sequence for Home Practice

Please take the night sequence slowly, taking your time and breath in each pose. You may use pillows or other props to help you support your body and relax.

Savasana with Breath and Body Awareness

◊ Begin by lying on your back, allowing your feet to fall to the sides while you release your hands, draw the arms out to the side, bending them at the elbows in cactus. Take a few moments to close your eyes and breath.

◊ Feel a sense of freedom spreading throughout your entire body.

◊ Draw both your knees in toward your chest, hug them and roll from side-to-side on your back.

Twists on Your Back

◊ Drop your knees to the right (while maintaining both your shoulders on the mat) and hold the twist for several breaths. Return to the center.

◊ Repeat the twist by dropping your knees to the left.
◊ Hug your knees in toward your chest and roll onto the right side of your body in a fetal position.

Wide Knee Child Pose

◊ Move from fetal position to kneeling. Widen your knees to the sides of the mat and relax your body between them, arms stretched in front of you and forehead on the floor in wide knee child pose.
◊ Hold wide knee child pose for several breaths.

Table-Top Sequence

◊ Move from your child pose to a table-top position. Draw your right hand under your body and twist towards the left. Breathe and move back to a table-top position.
◊ Repeat by drawing your left hand under your body and twist to your right.
◊ After returning to a neutral table-top position, release back to a child pose

Pigeon

◊ Move from child pose back to neutral table-top position.
◊ Send your right knee forward, your shin parallel with the front edge of your mat and your left leg extended behind you, and take pigeon pose on the right side.
◊ Slowly release from pigeon to child pose.

◊ Repeat the other side by moving to a neutral table and sending your left leg forward to a pigeon pose. Return to child pose when you're ready.

◊ From child pose, move to a comfortable seated position with both legs straight forward and forward fold for several breaths (*paschimottanasana*).

Move to Lie on Your Back

◊ From your seated forward fold move gently to lie on your back, drawing your feet together and spreading your knees apart in *baddha konasana*.

◊ Place your hands on your lower belly and follow your breath.

Legs up the Wall

◊ Move to a wall, sitting with your hips and back to the wall.

◊ When you're ready hug your knees in toward your chest and roll to fetal position.

◊ From fetal position, gently move your legs up the wall, straightening them incrementally.

◊ Hold for five to seven minutes.

Savasana

◊ Gently hug your knees to your chest and carefully move away from the wall.

◊ Place a pillow under your knees or under your legs in a manner that's extremely comfortable in order to move to a supported savasana.

◊ Lay on your back. Relax every part of your body. Focus on your shoulders, then your arms, then your hands, and so on.

◊ Stay in savasana for as long as your body wants or needs.

Good night!

Meditation

Instructions for a simple home meditation.

◊ First, if possible, find a suitable place where you feel comfortable.

◊ Find a comfortable seated position. Close your eyes. Take a few moments to adjust yourself so you can find a comfortable position where you'll be able to stay relatively still as you meditate.

◊ Center your sitting bones and pelvis. Lengthen your torso gently. Keep your chest open but relaxed. Soften your jaw, allow the tongue to rest at the bottom of the mouth. Relax your lips.

◊ Place your palms on your thighs with a light touch. Return to your breath. When ready, if you want to, according to the Shamata Buddhist school of thought, you may lightly open your eyes softly looking downwards. Glance downward at a spot several feet away from the tip of your nose. If you prefer, you may keep your eyes shut. Find what works best for you.

◊ Notice your breath moving in your body. Don't try to alter or change it. Simply observe your natural pattern of breath. Return to your breath again and again as your point of attention.

◊ As random thoughts arise, and they will, simply return to the breath, again and again.

◊ Imagine your breath as a bench that you will return to sit on again and again. Every time a thought rises up, return your attention to your breath as if you stood up and are returning to the bench to sit down again.

◊ Sit for a few minutes or more. Allow space for everything that comes up with no judgment or aggression. Have a gentle approach toward yourself.

◊ Take your hands in prayer in front of your heart center, allowing yourself to complete your seated meditation.

◊ When you feel ready, gently and carefully exit your seated position and continue forward with your day or night.

Resources

Bibliography

Brown, Brené. *Atlas of the Heart*. New York, NY: Random House, 2021.

Chödrön, Pema.

"How to Practice Tonglen." Lion's Roar: Buddhist Widsom for Our Time. January 1, 2023. https://www.lionsroar.com/how-to-practice-tonglen/.

Living Beautifully: with Uncertainty and Change. Boulder, CO: Shambhala, 2012.

The Places That Scare You. Boulder, CO: Shambhala, 2007.

The Pocket Pema Chödrön. Boulder, CO: Shambhala, 2008.

When Things Fall Apart. Boulder, CO: Shambhala, 1996.

The Wisdom of No Escape and the Path of Loving-Kindness. Boulder, CO: Shambhala, 2001.

Daishonin, Nichiren. "Buddhism: Overcome Your Arrogance." Nichiren Shoshu Myosenji Buddhist Temple. July 2017. https://nstmyosenji.org/feelings-of-arrogance.

Hanh, Thich Nhat. *The Art of Living*. London, England: Penguin Random House UK, 2017.

Iyengar, B. K. S. *Light on Yoga*. N.p: Schocken Books, 1979.

Mehta, Silva, Shyam Mehta, and Mira Mehta. Yoga: The Iyengar Way. New York, NY: Alfred A. Knopf, 1990.

Mipham, Sakyong. "Make Your Decisions for Others." Lion's Roar. Last modified July 1, 2004. Accessed October 13, 2023. https://www.lionsroar.com/make-your-decisions-for-others/.

Satchidananda, Sri Swami. *The Yoga Sutras of Patanjali.* Compiled by Patanjali. N.p.: Integral Yoga Publications, 1990.

Recommended Reading

If you would like to study the precepts of yoga and meditation, I recommend beginning with these works that I feel are accessible to everyone regardless of background or depth of knowledge:

- ◊ *The Yoga Sutras of Patanjali* by Satchidananda and Patanjali
- ◊ *When Things Fall Apart* by Pema Chödrön
- ◊ *Light on Yoga* by B.K.S. Iyengar

Acknowledgements

The challenge of writing a book has been an eye-opening experience where I've learned so much and keep realizing that I've just scratched the surface of what I need to know. The first lesson I learned was that writing a book is simultaneously a very personal, private affair, but it's equally a team effort. It's a titanic effort that depends on the hard work, vision, dedication, and belief of a large group of people. Here I want to attempt to acknowledge all the people without whose efforts, this book would not exist.

I want to thank my husband Jonathan, who put in countless hours of work to make sure the book became a reality, and my children Nadav, Netta, and Romi, who provided inspiration, wisdom, and ideas, and without whom I could never have written the book.

I must thank my dear friend Hadas Weisman, who generously, on her own initiative, shared my manuscript with my publisher. Her thoughtfulness represented a key turning point, without which the book would never have been published.

Of course, I need to thank the entire team at How2Conquer. Their creativity and professionalism helped raise the quality of the final product to a whole new level, which truly captured my voice and my vision. In our first Zoom call together, Michelle Newcome immediately used the design from a panel she saw behind me as the inspiration for the style of the cover and artwork. I must thank Charlotte Bleau and Lauren Kelliher for their amazing editing work and for graciously answering all my questions, and of course, Telia Garner for both the brilliant illustrations and her work as part of the editing team.

I need to thank my students, who comprise the wonderful community at my yoga studio. They are a joy to work with. They motivate and inspire me daily to be a better teacher and person, to keep learning and developing myself, and to keep giving back.

Everyone here, and many others, have played a role in this endeavor, and I want to thank all of them.

Danit Schreiber

About Danit

Danit Schreiber has been teaching and continuing to study yoga and meditation for over fifteen years and has taught thousands of hours of classes. Over this time, Danit has developed a unique voice and her own distinctive style of teaching which has evolved into the Yoga By Danit Method™. Danit's method focuses on achieving the greatest opening of the body and mind through a combination of effort and surrender. Uniting proper breathing with movement helps students attain the level of relaxation needed to open energy flow in the body to both strengthen and stretch their muscles and calm their mind. The method extends beyond the classroom and endeavors to provide students with practical tools they can use to improve the quality of their day-to-day lives. The studio she founded has become a special community where students feel mutually supported, empowered, and safe, a place where they're inspired to face the challenges of modern life.

Danit has been practicing yoga and meditation on a daily basis for many years. She finds yoga to be a natural extension of her long-time experience as a ballet dancer. During her years of teaching, Danit has achieved the certification level of E-RYT 500 and YACEP. Certified in vinyasa, restorative, yin, meditation (Reiki healing, baby and me, and postpartum yoga). Danit is constantly studying, refreshing, and expanding her knowledge, taking courses beyond yoga certification including anatomy and the science of stretching.

Danit provides students with a broad range of possibilities and approaches. Her method balances a focus on strong alignment and precise movements with mind and breath awareness that enables her students to both work and rejuvenate. Her classes are built on creative sequencing and a unique style to awaken and evoke the students' physical and mental awareness.

Prior to teaching Yoga, Danit worked in the business world. After serving in the Israeli Air Force, Danit completed her law degree and practiced as a litigator for several years in Tel Aviv. Danit worked as a corporate executive for several years before she and her family moved to the US.

In the US Danit started a successful business in teaching and presentation skills. Danit decided to pursue yoga because it gave her the satisfaction and joy of helping and supporting people in a manner that none of her previous endeavors could match. Being able to give people the same pleasure and benefits from yoga that Danit herself has enjoyed is the ultimate reward. The mother of three wonderful children, Danit lives with her husband in Rye, New York.

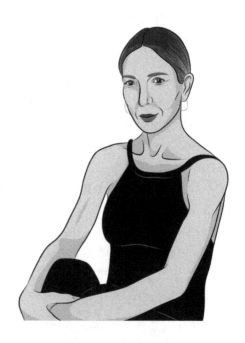

Printed in the USA
CPSIA information can be obtained
at www.ICGtesting.com
LVHW021607291123
764735LV00006B/34